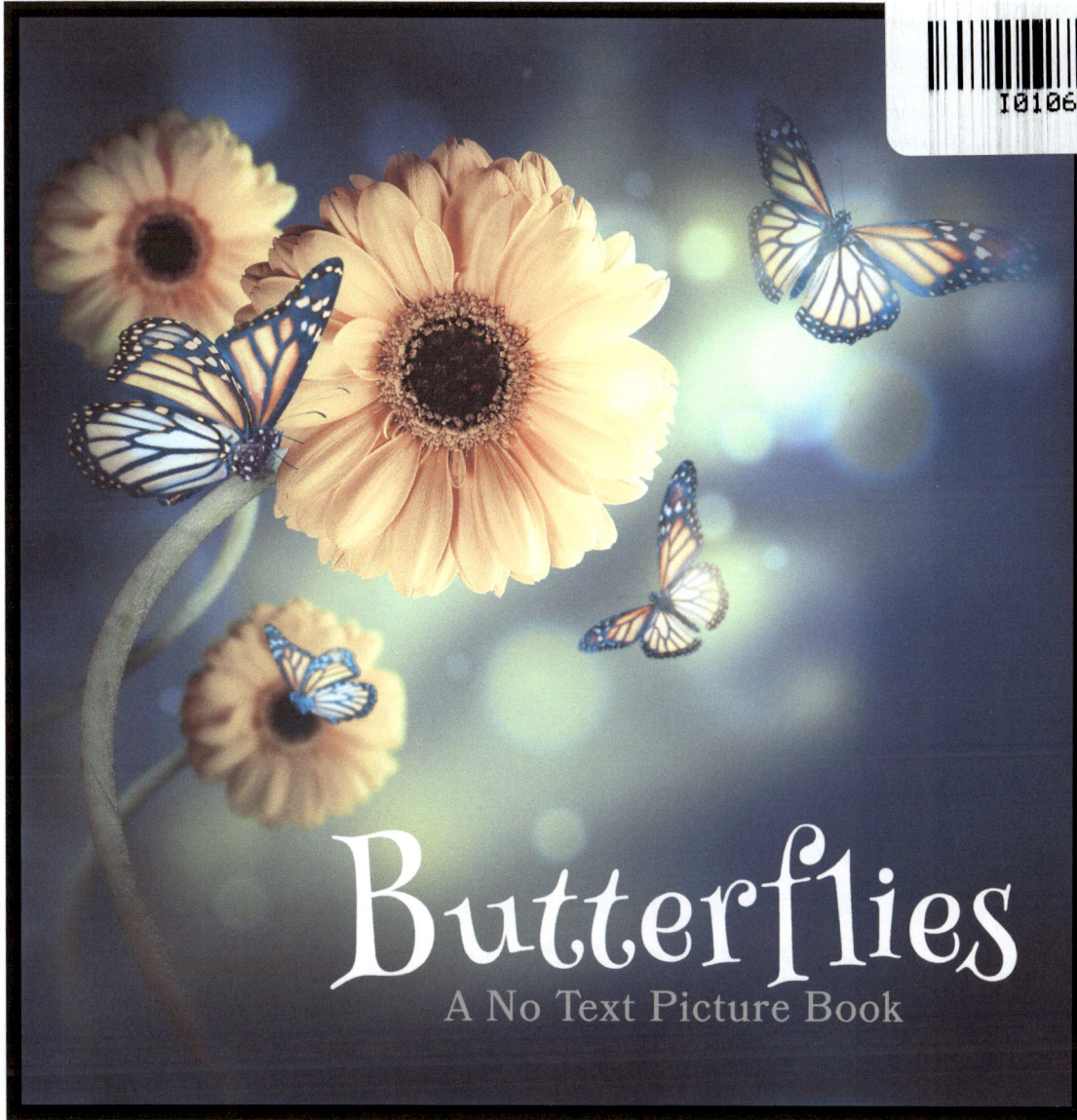

Butterflies
A No Text Picture Book

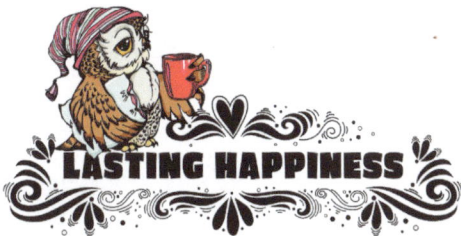

LASTING HAPPINESS

ISBN: 978-1-990181-17-7

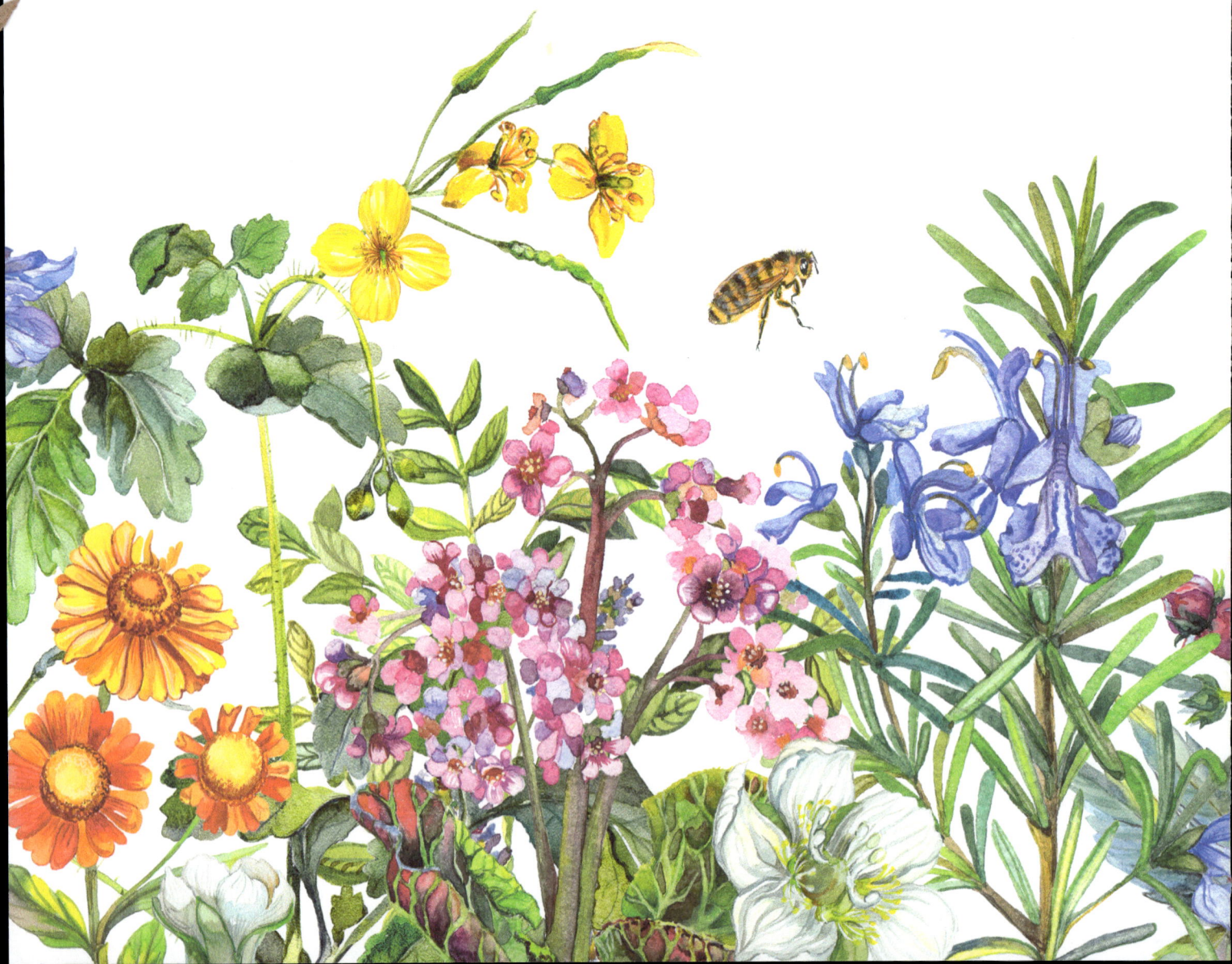

To:

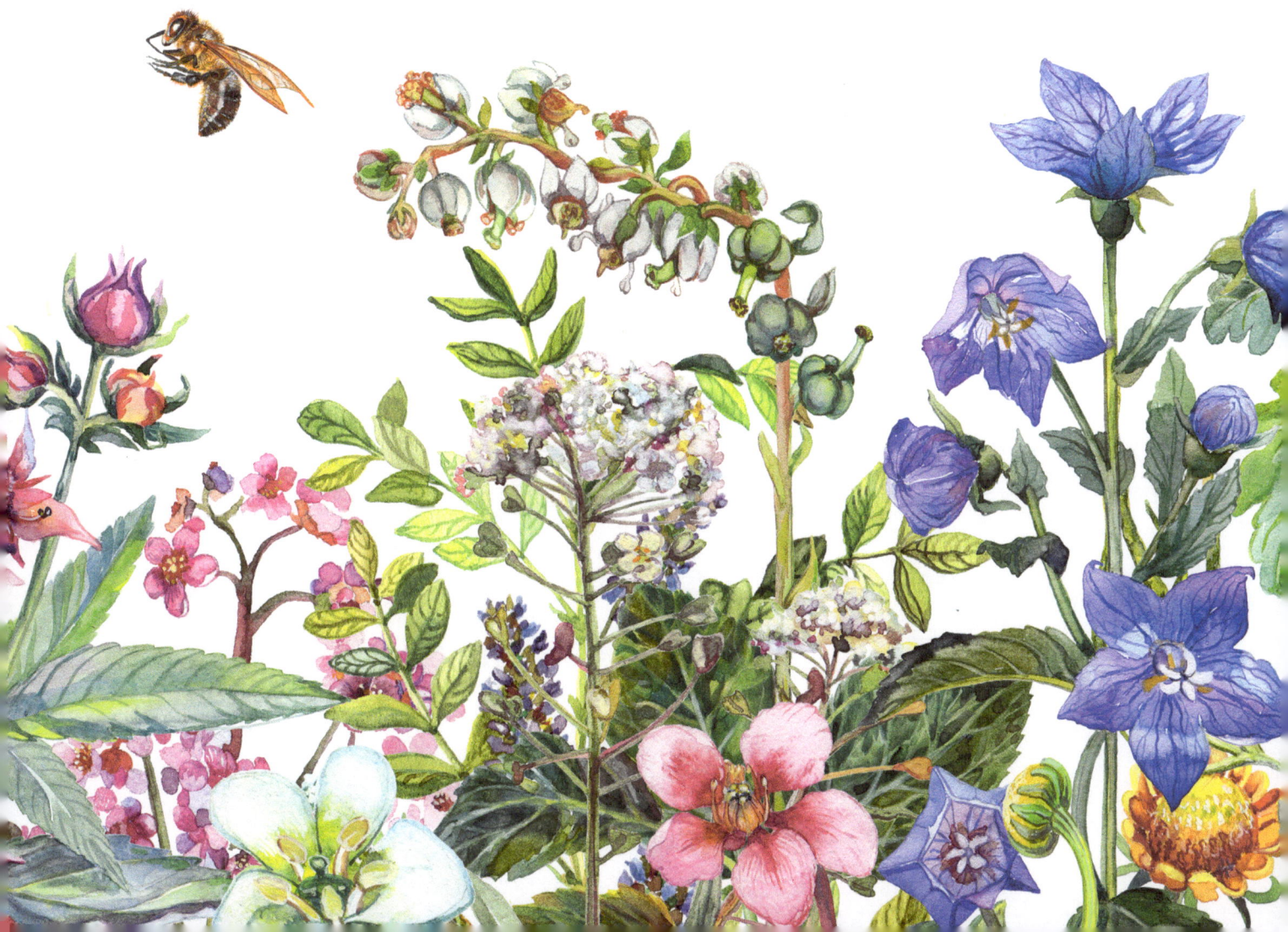

FROM:

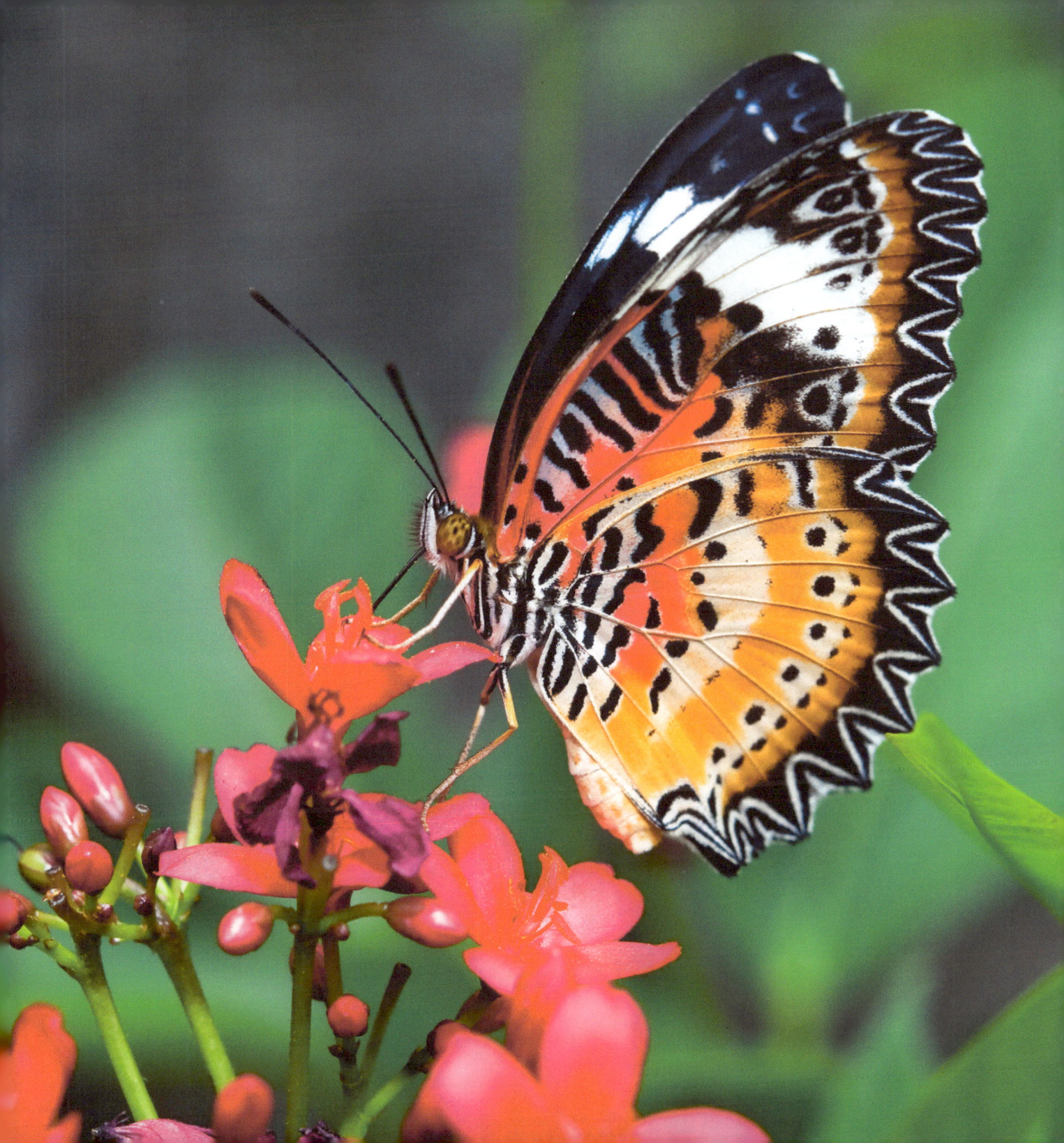

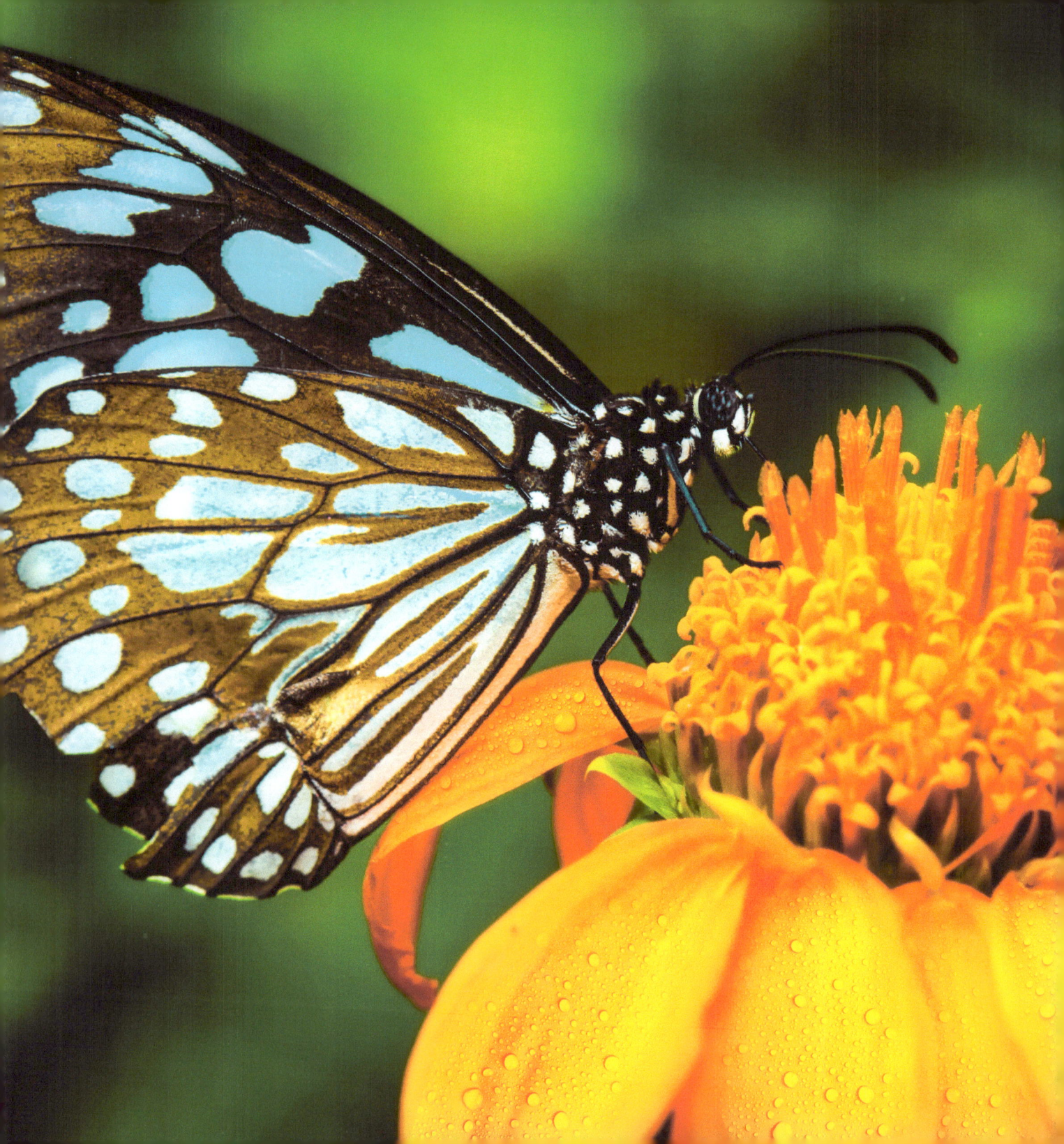

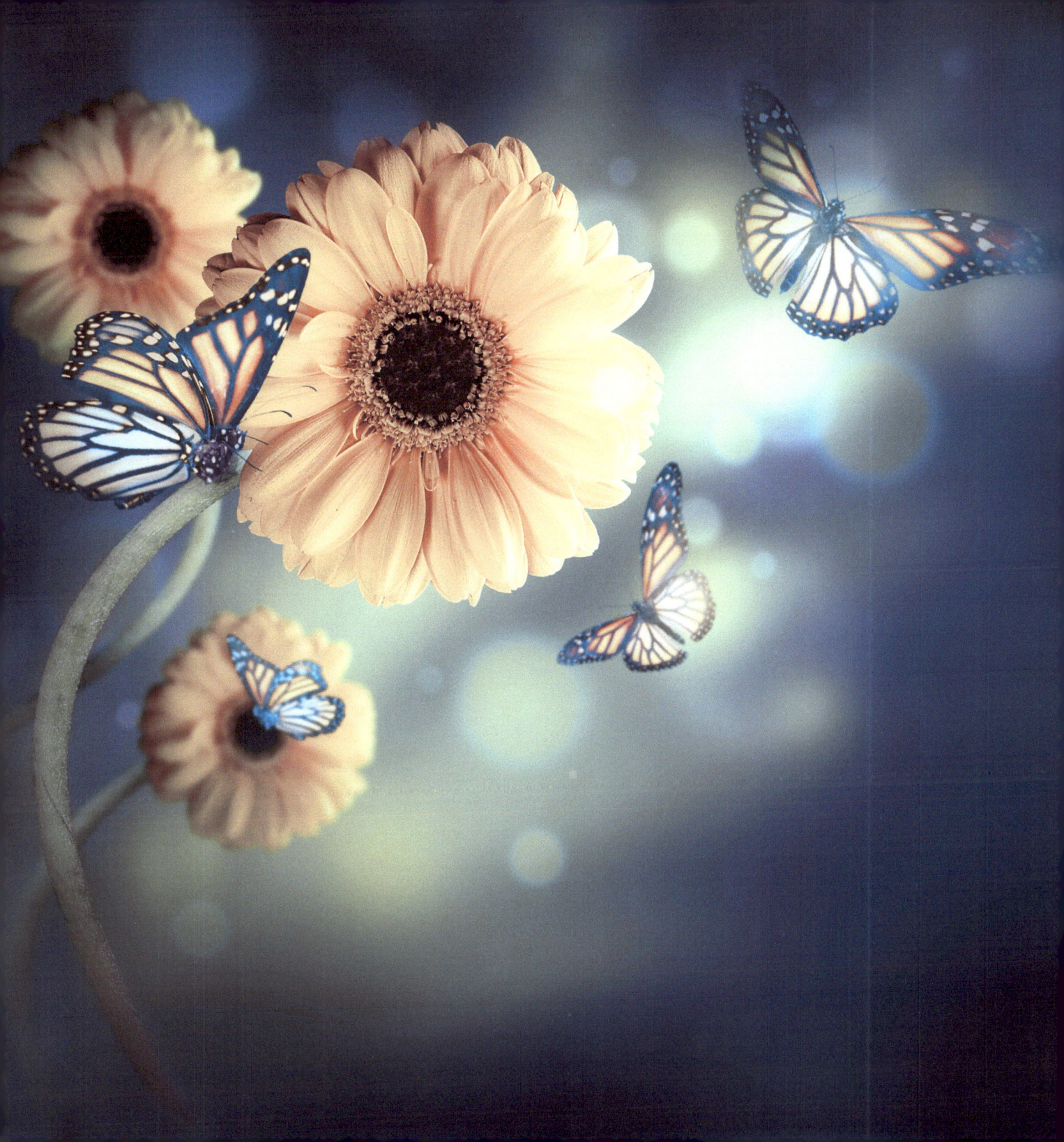

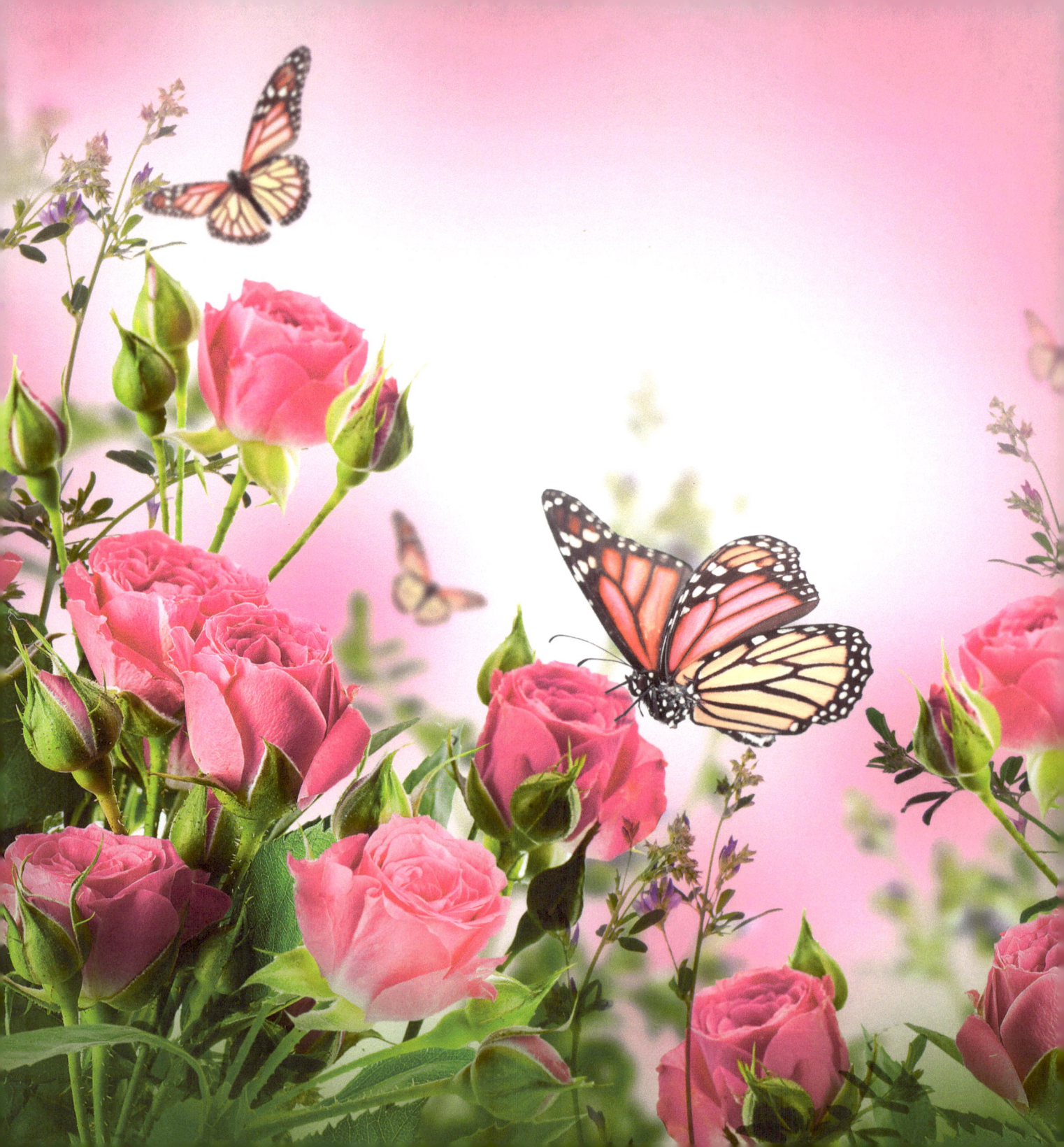

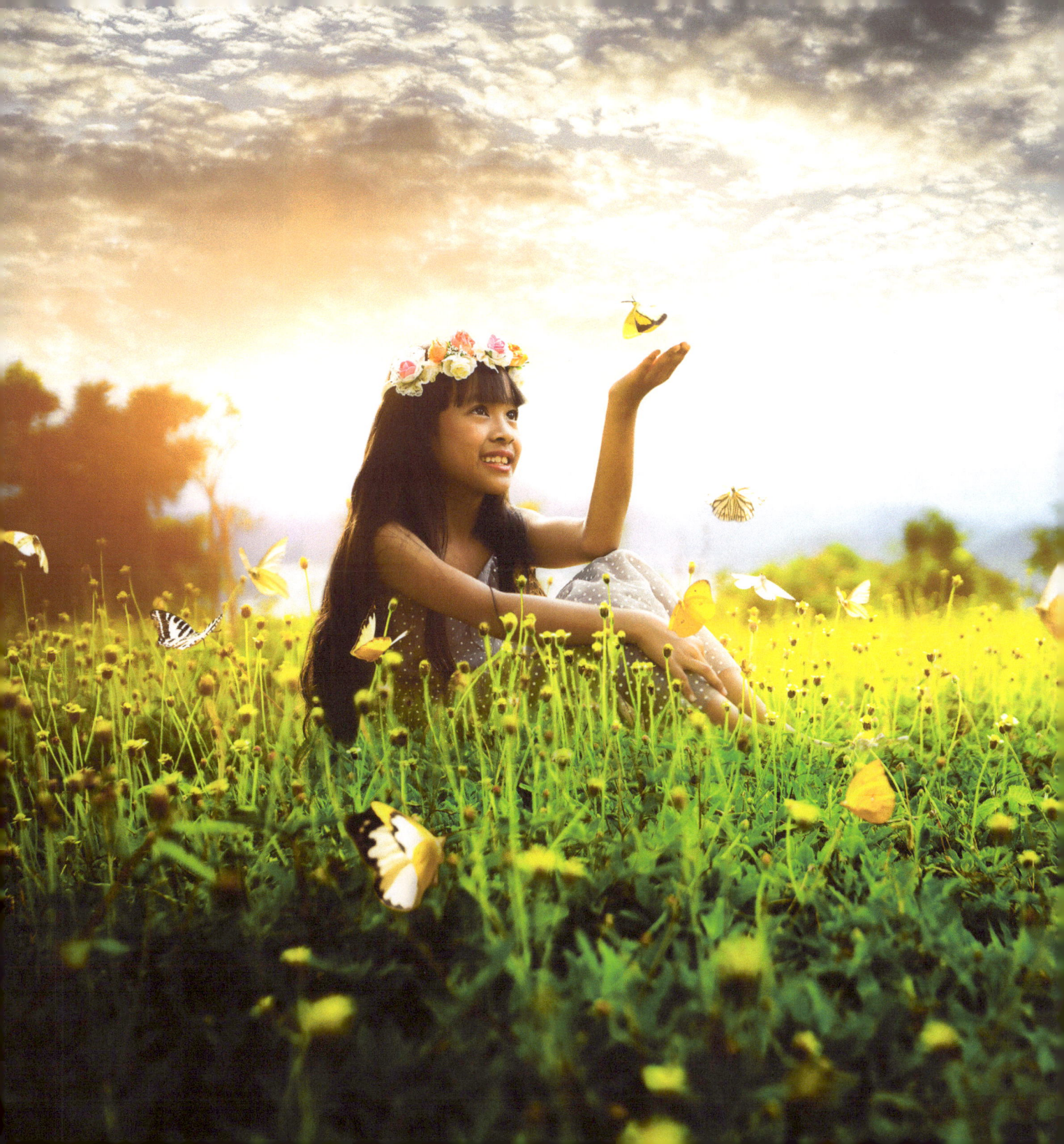

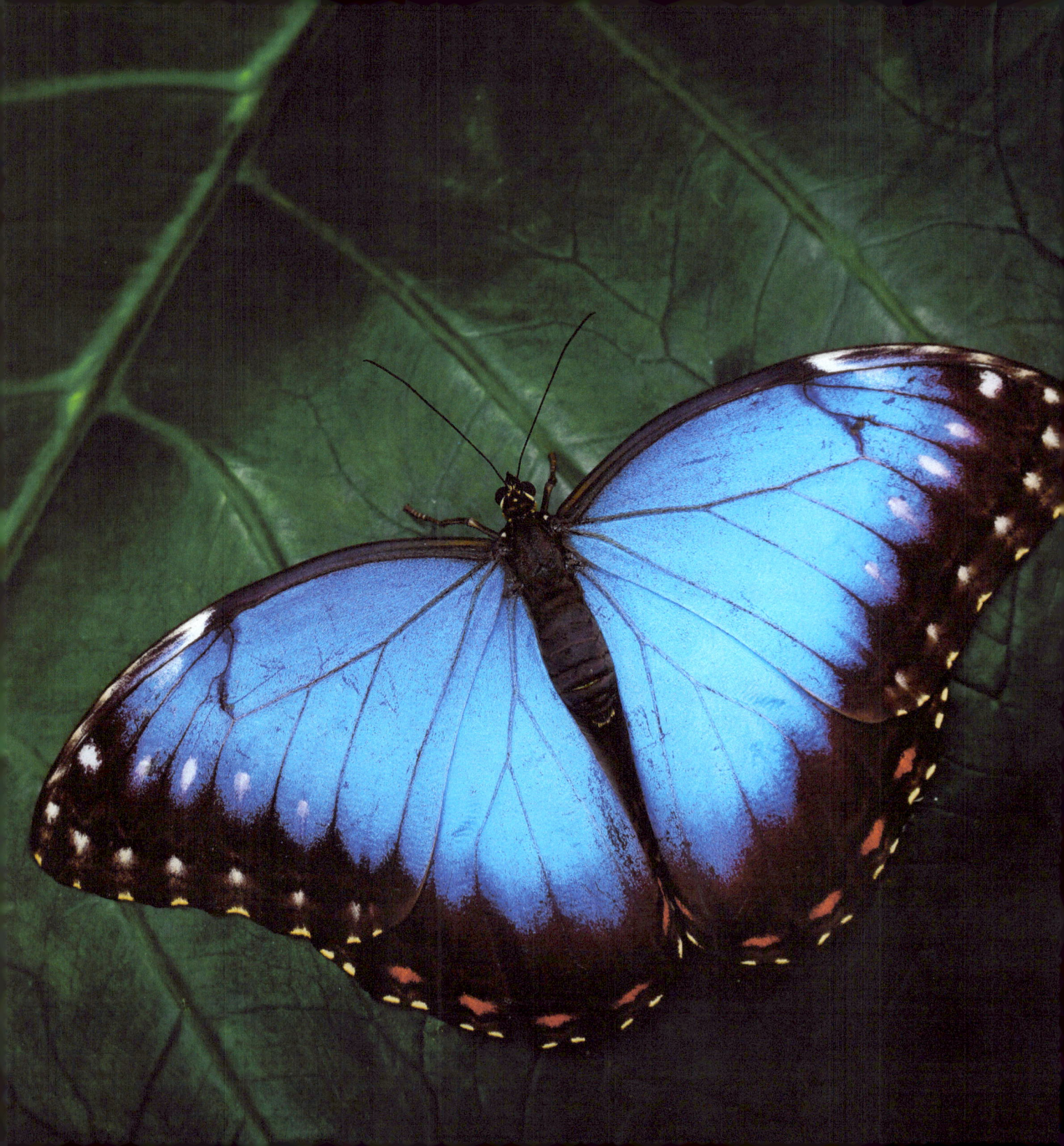

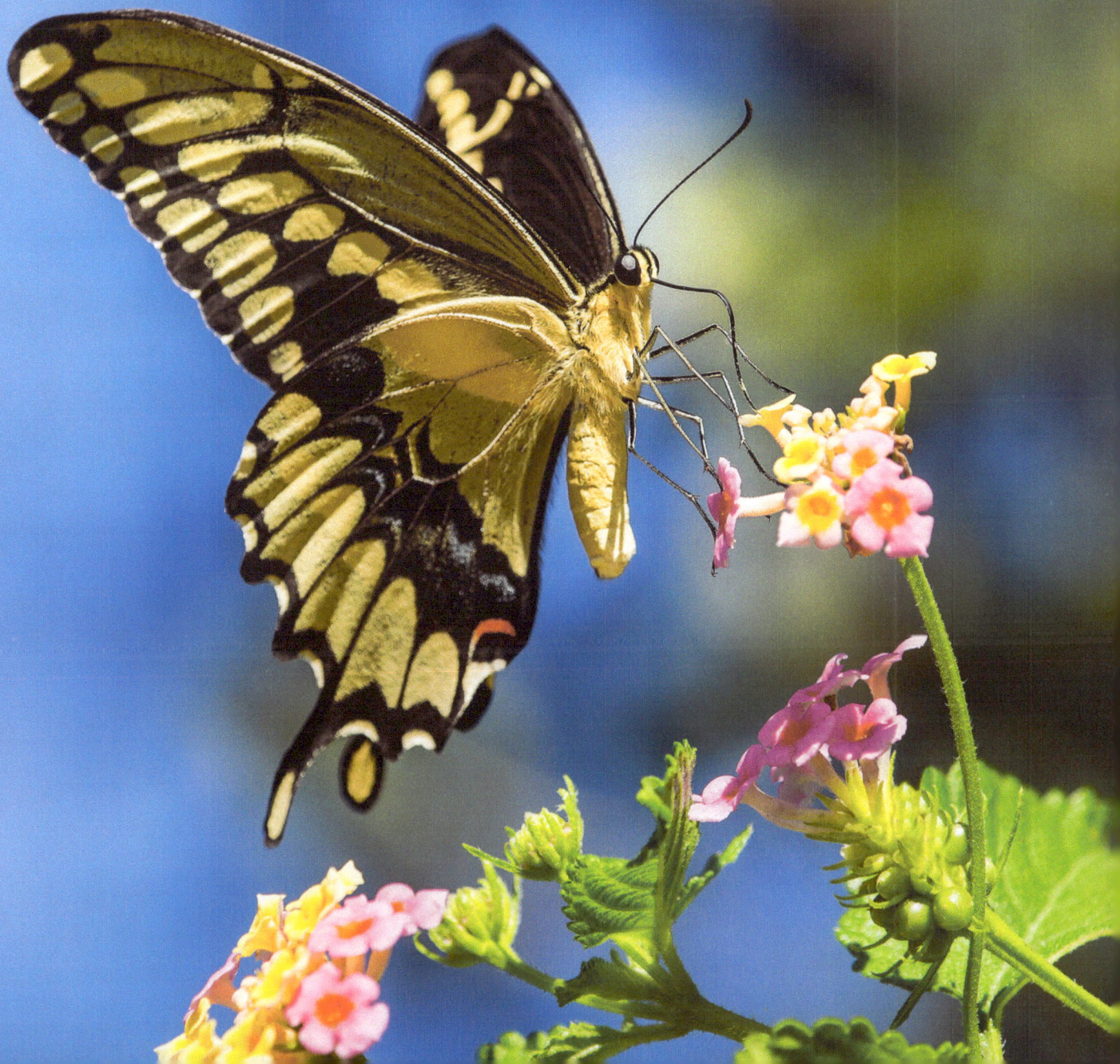

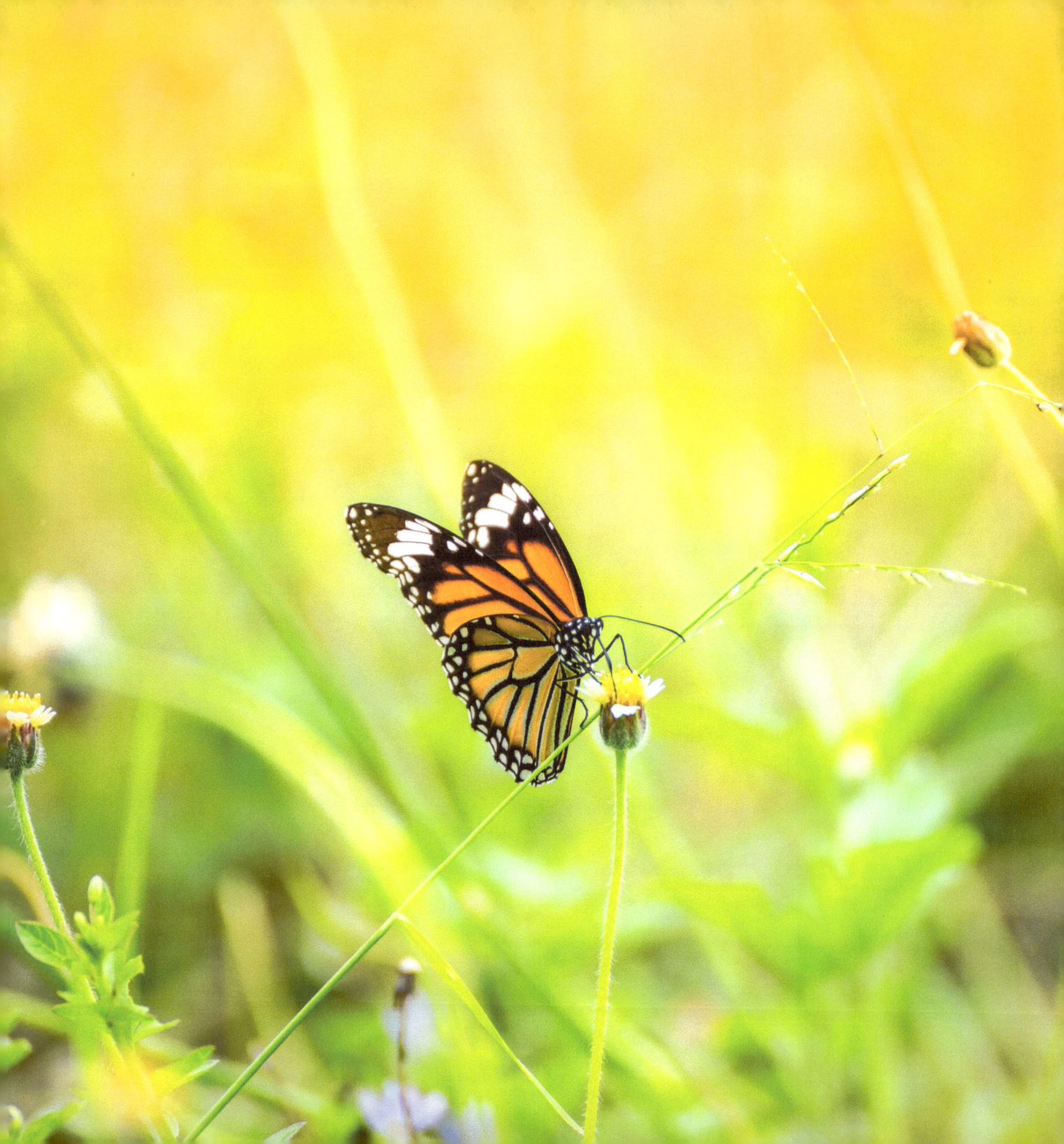

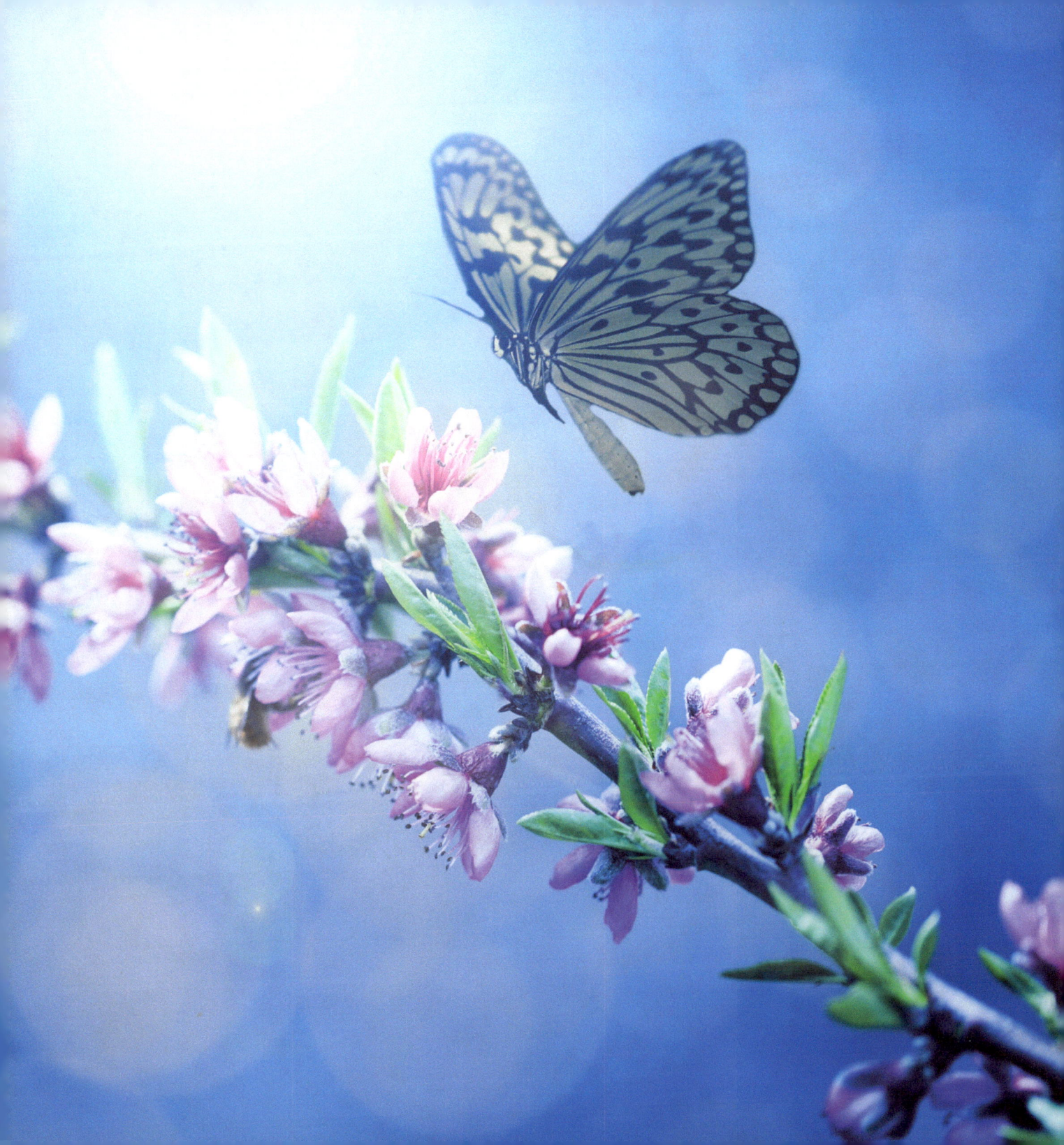

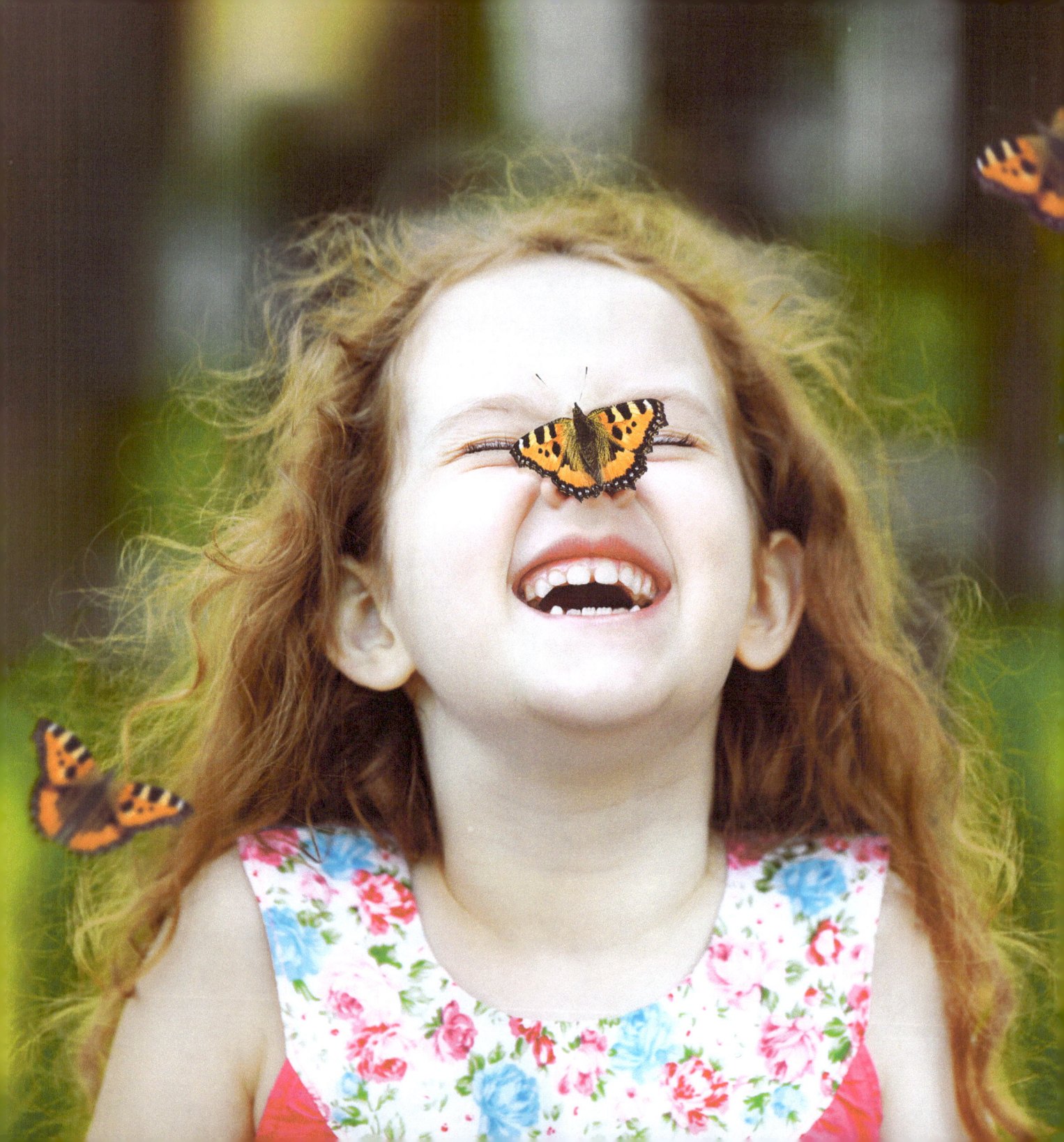

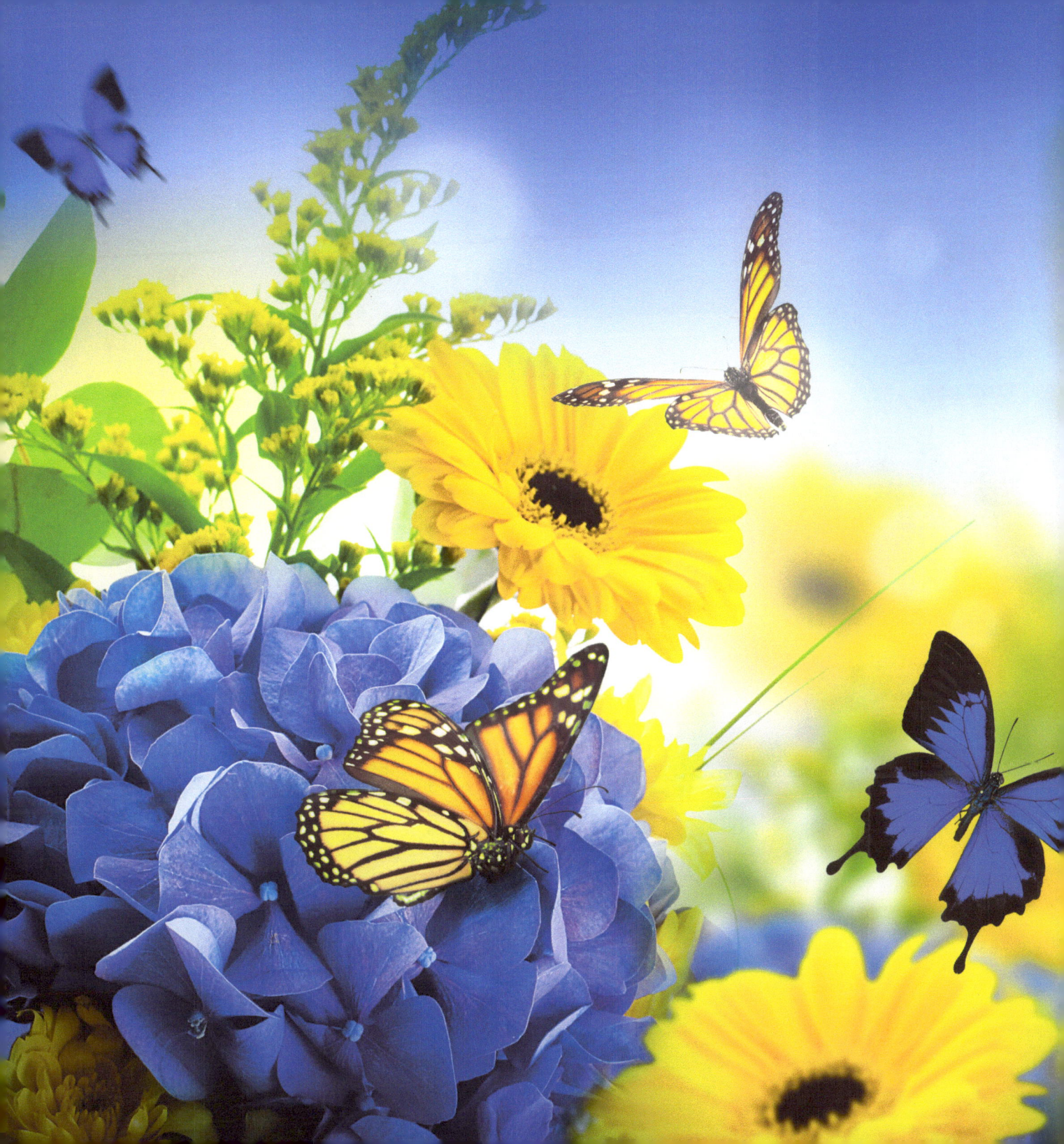

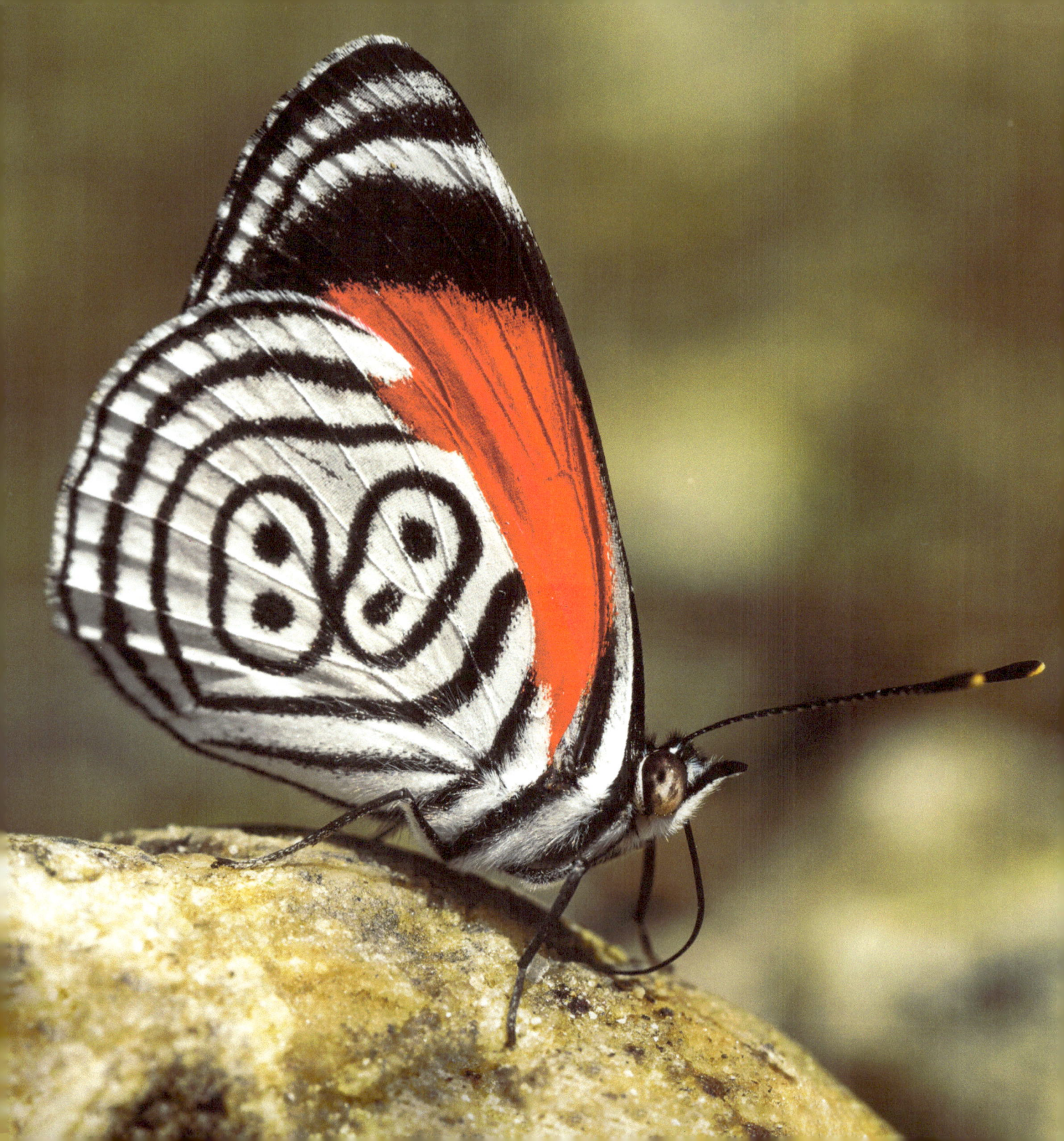

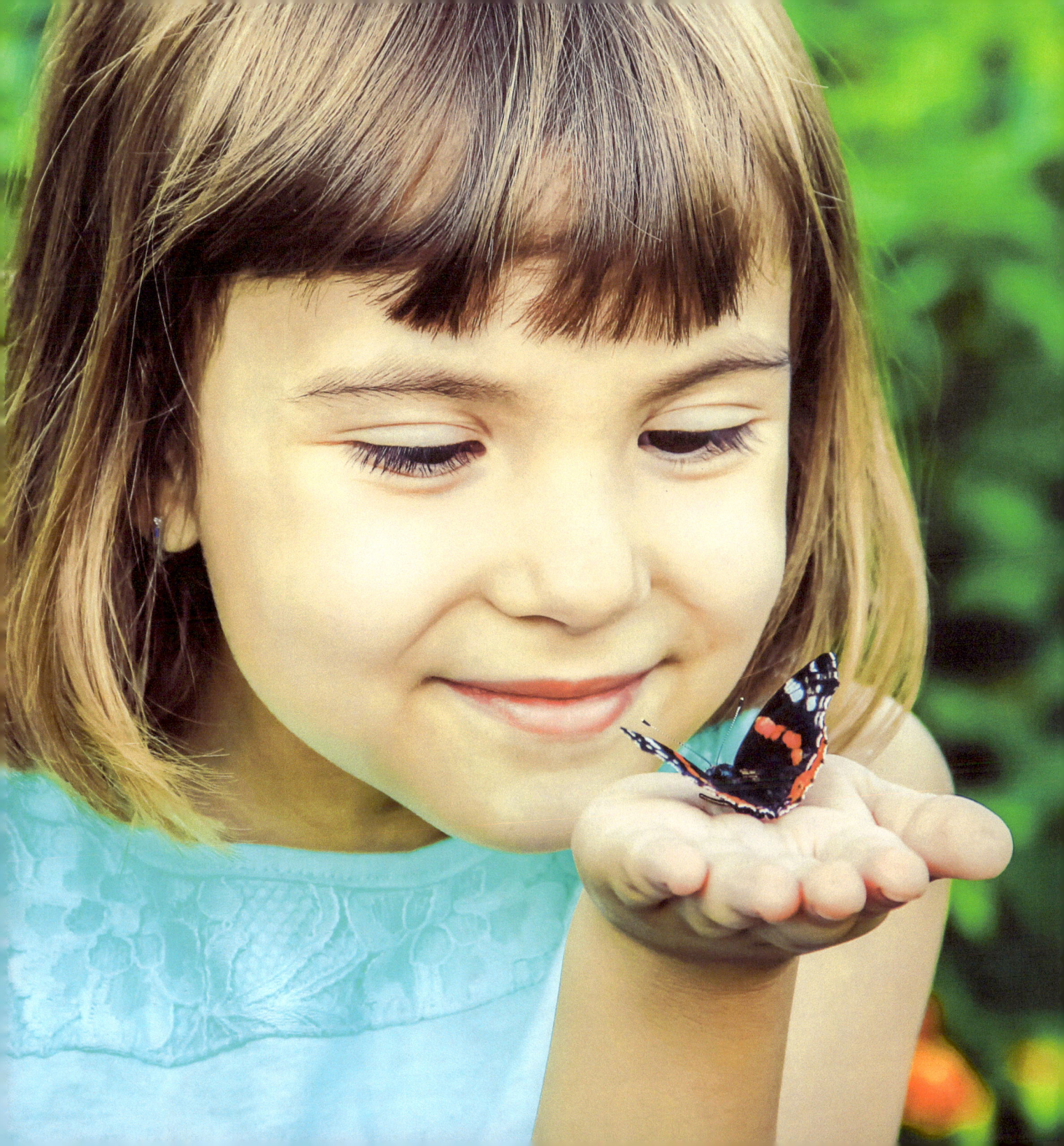

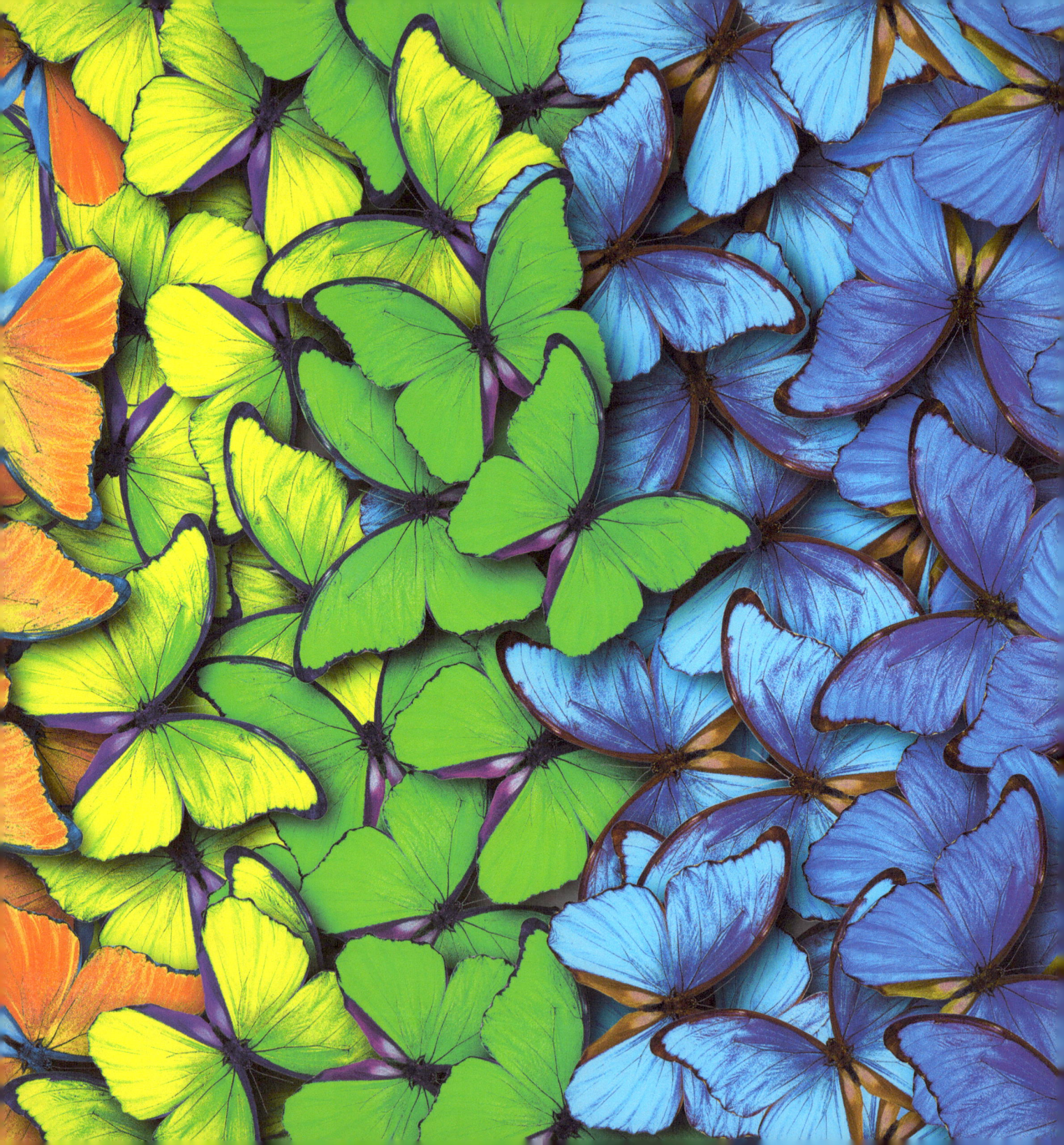

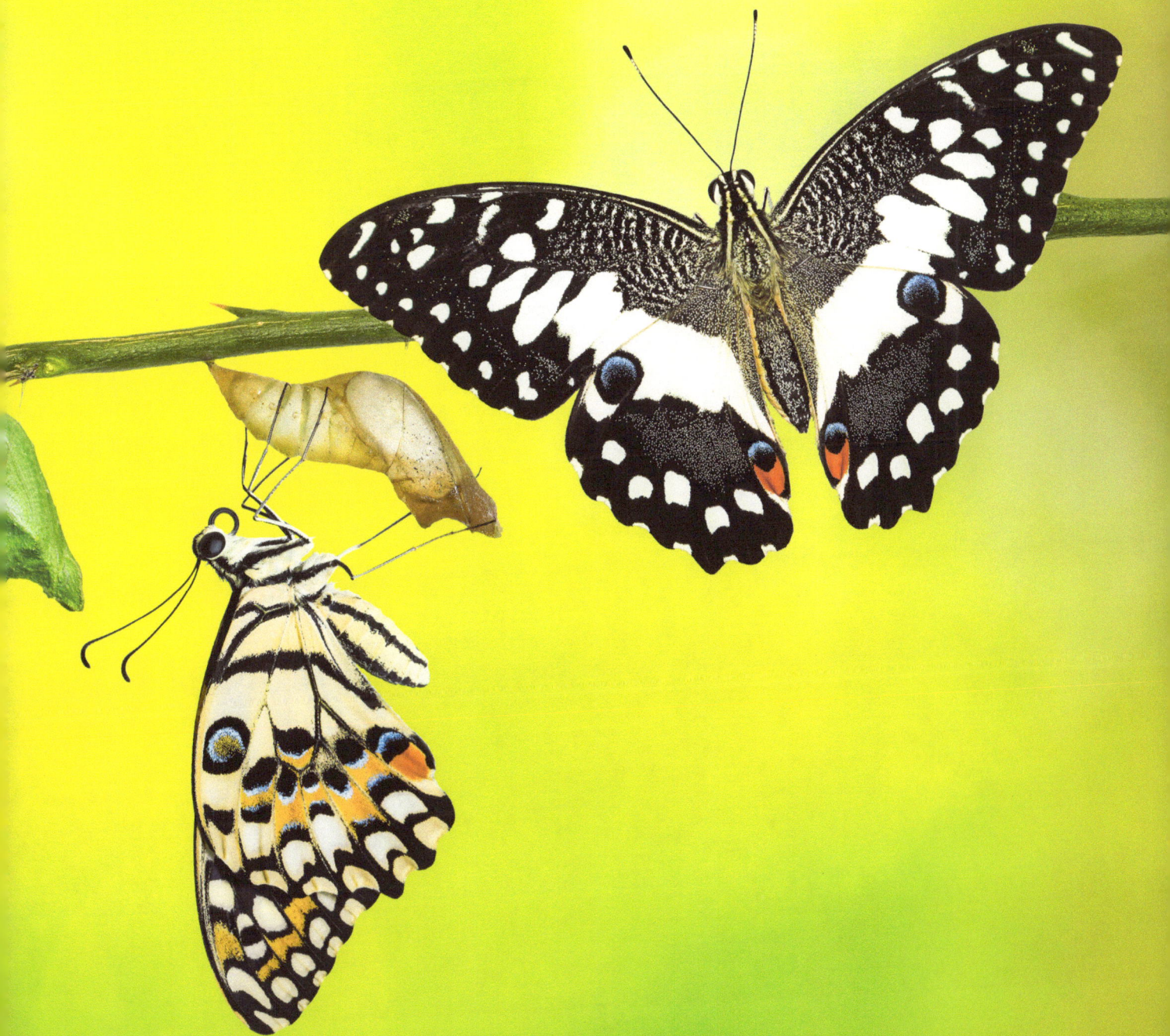

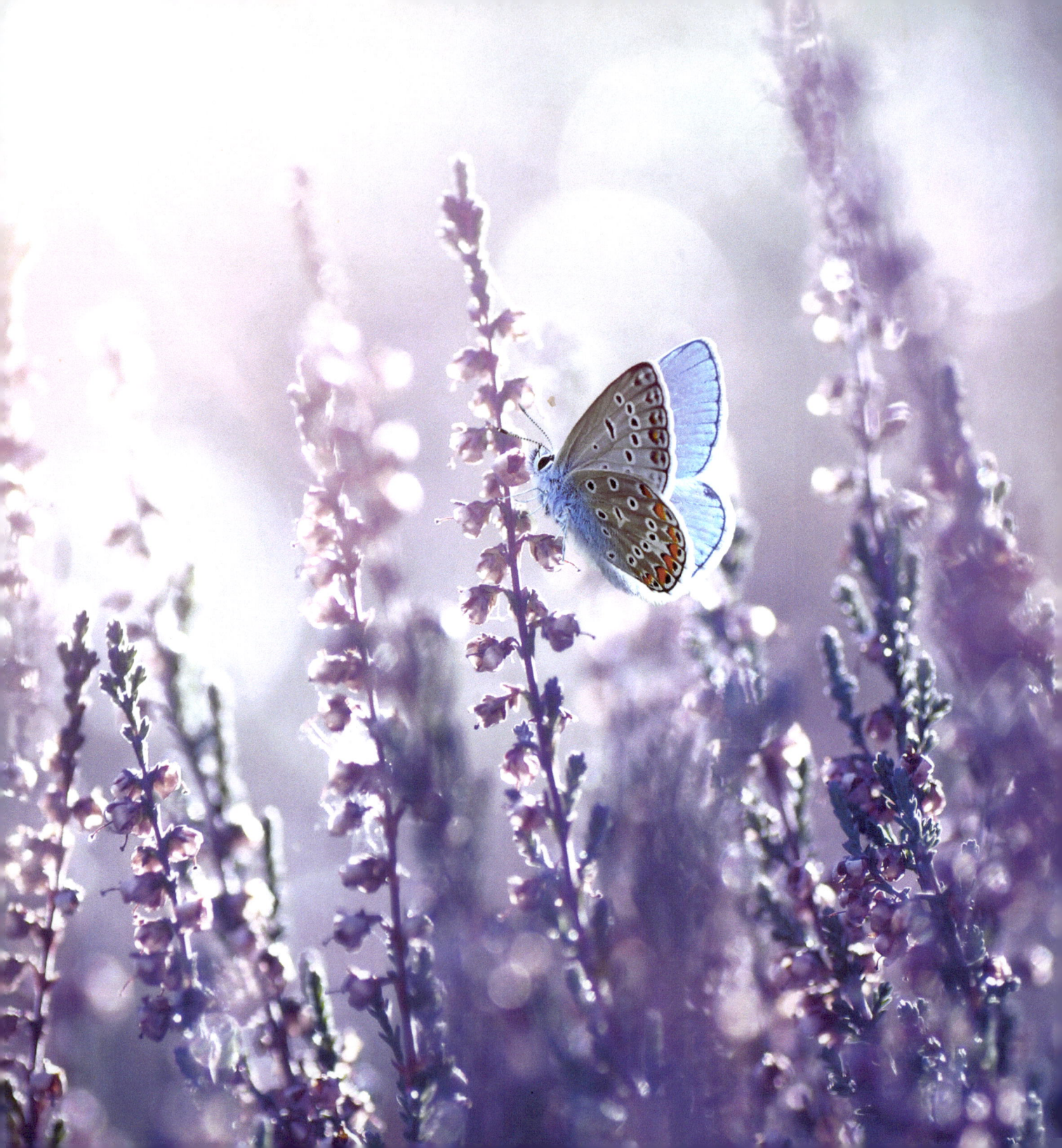

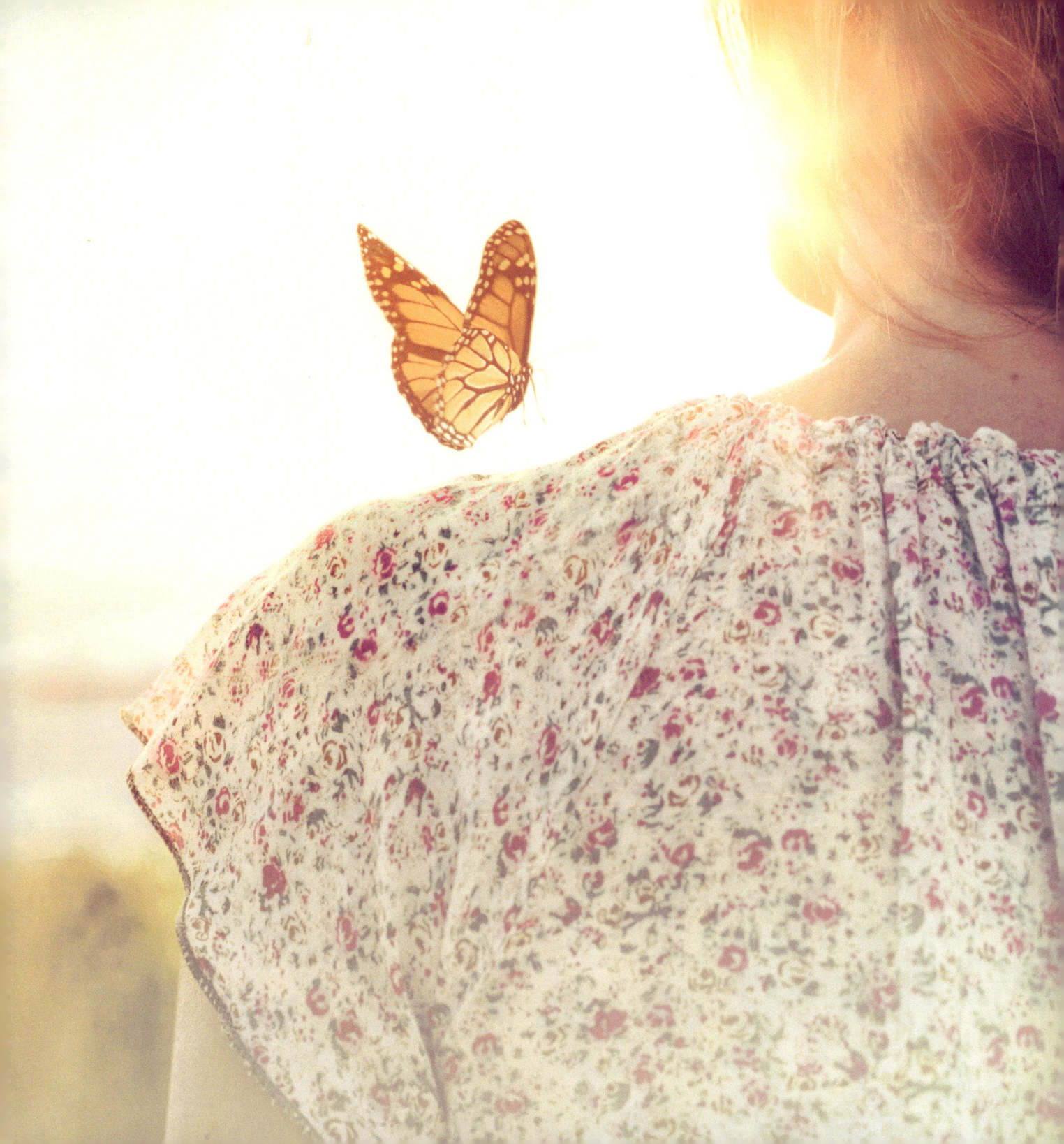

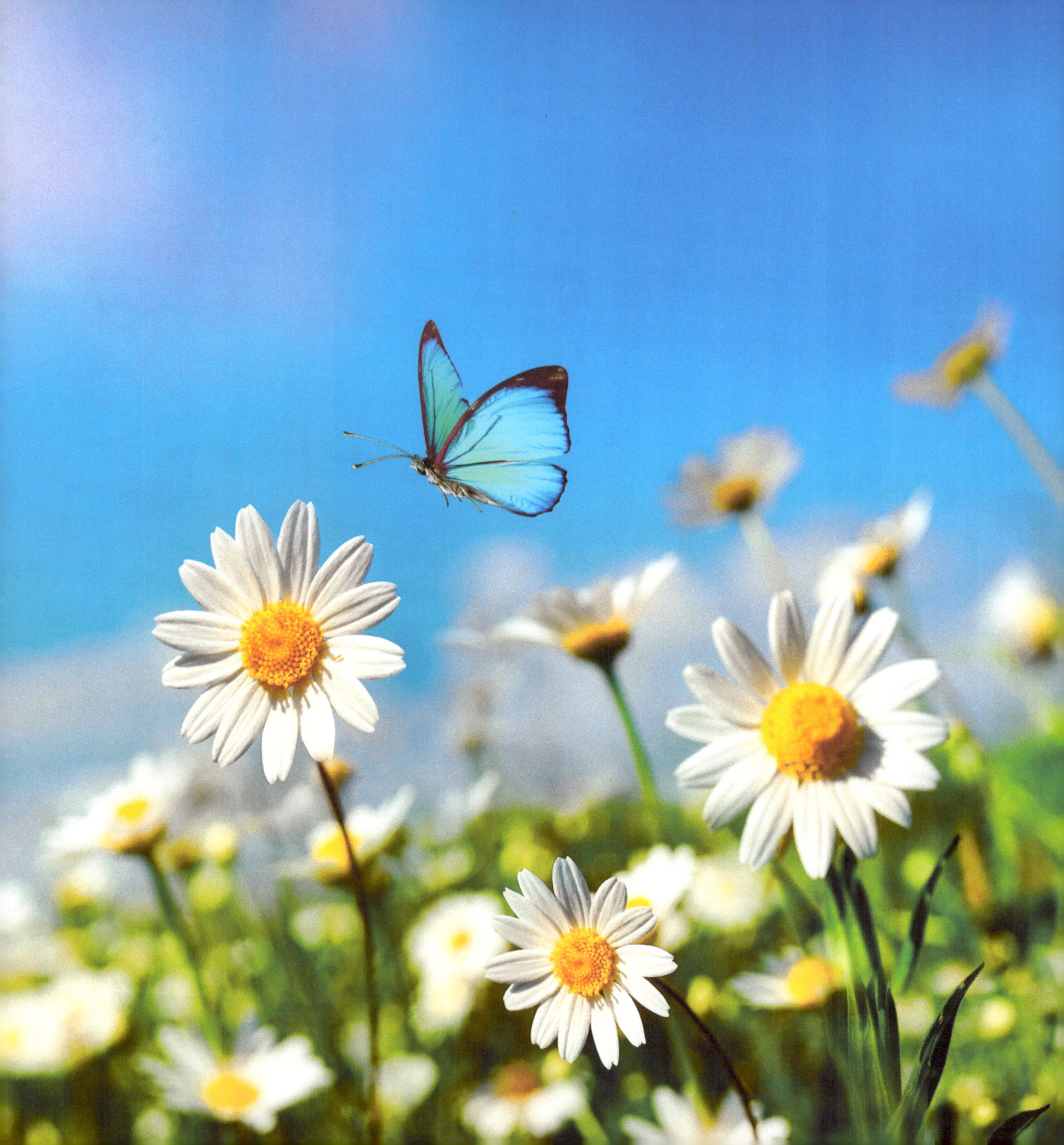

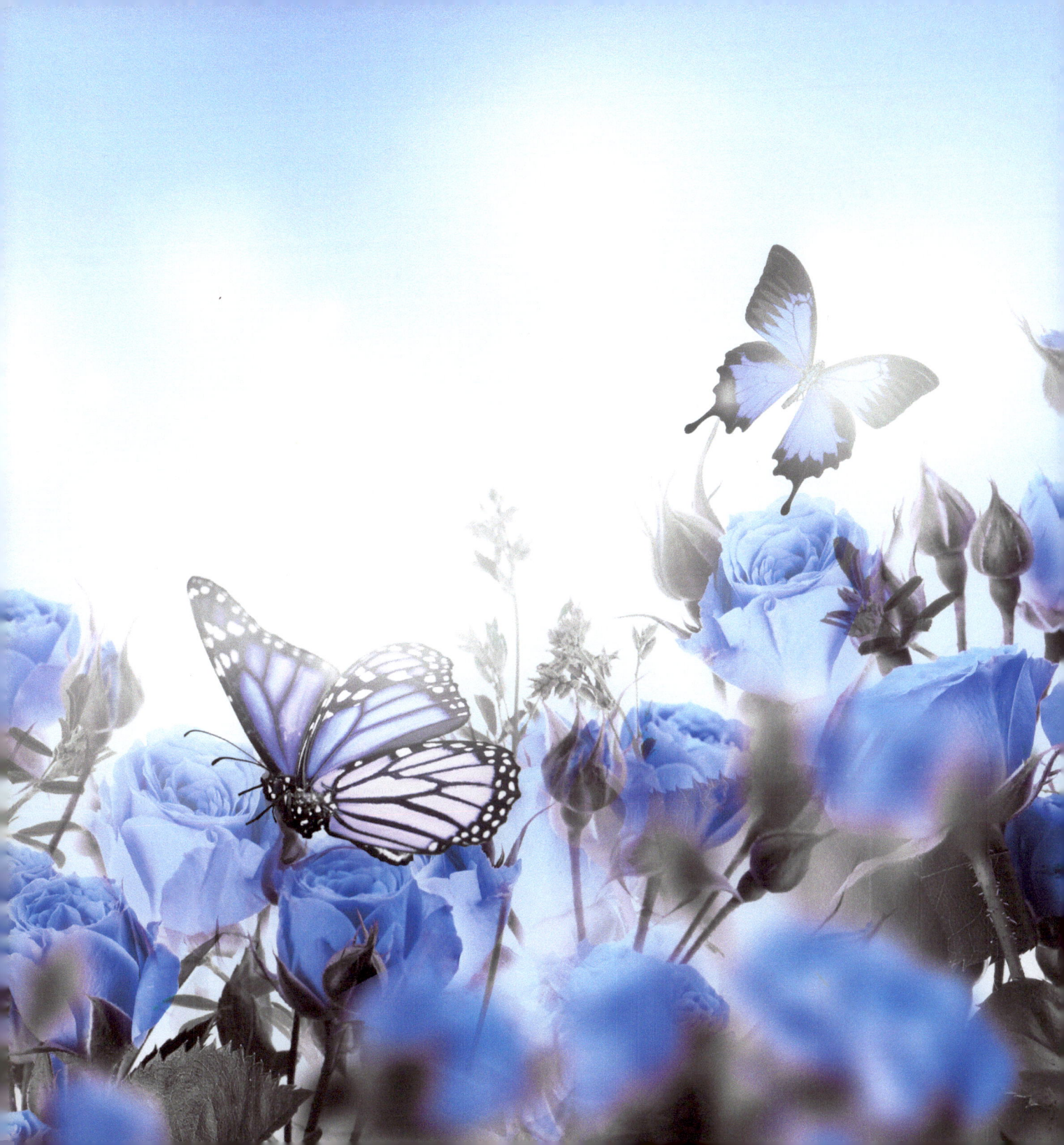

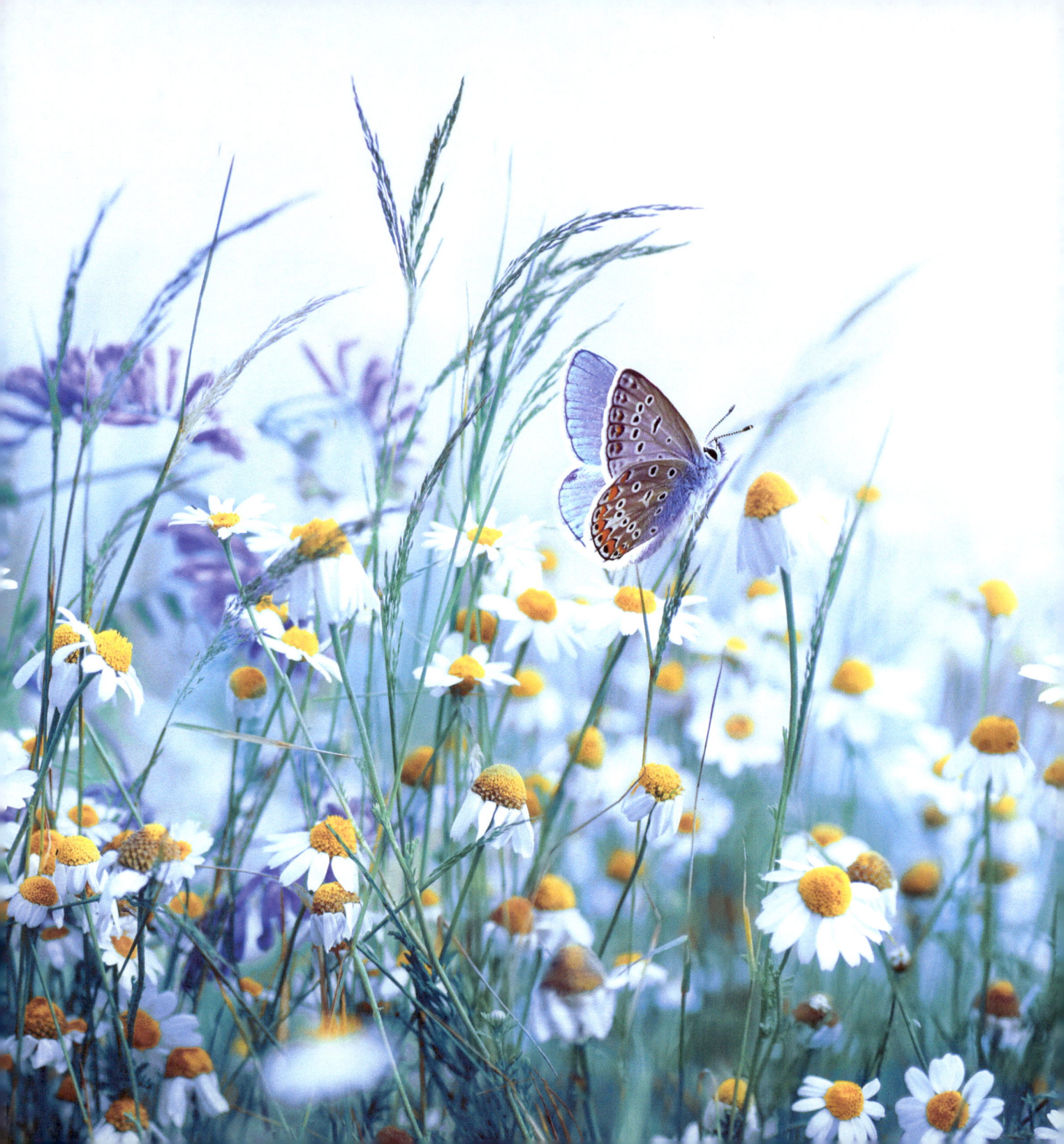

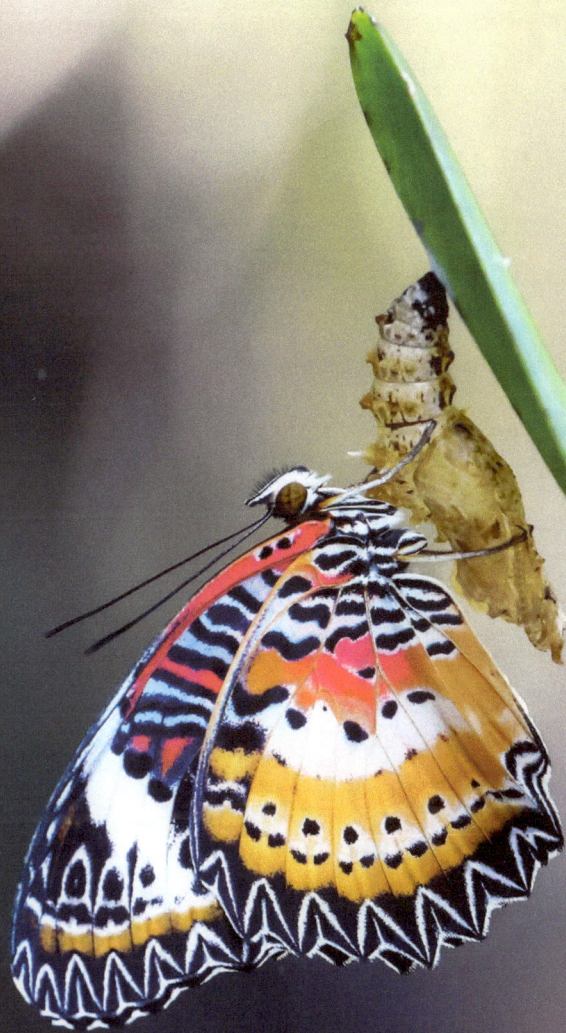

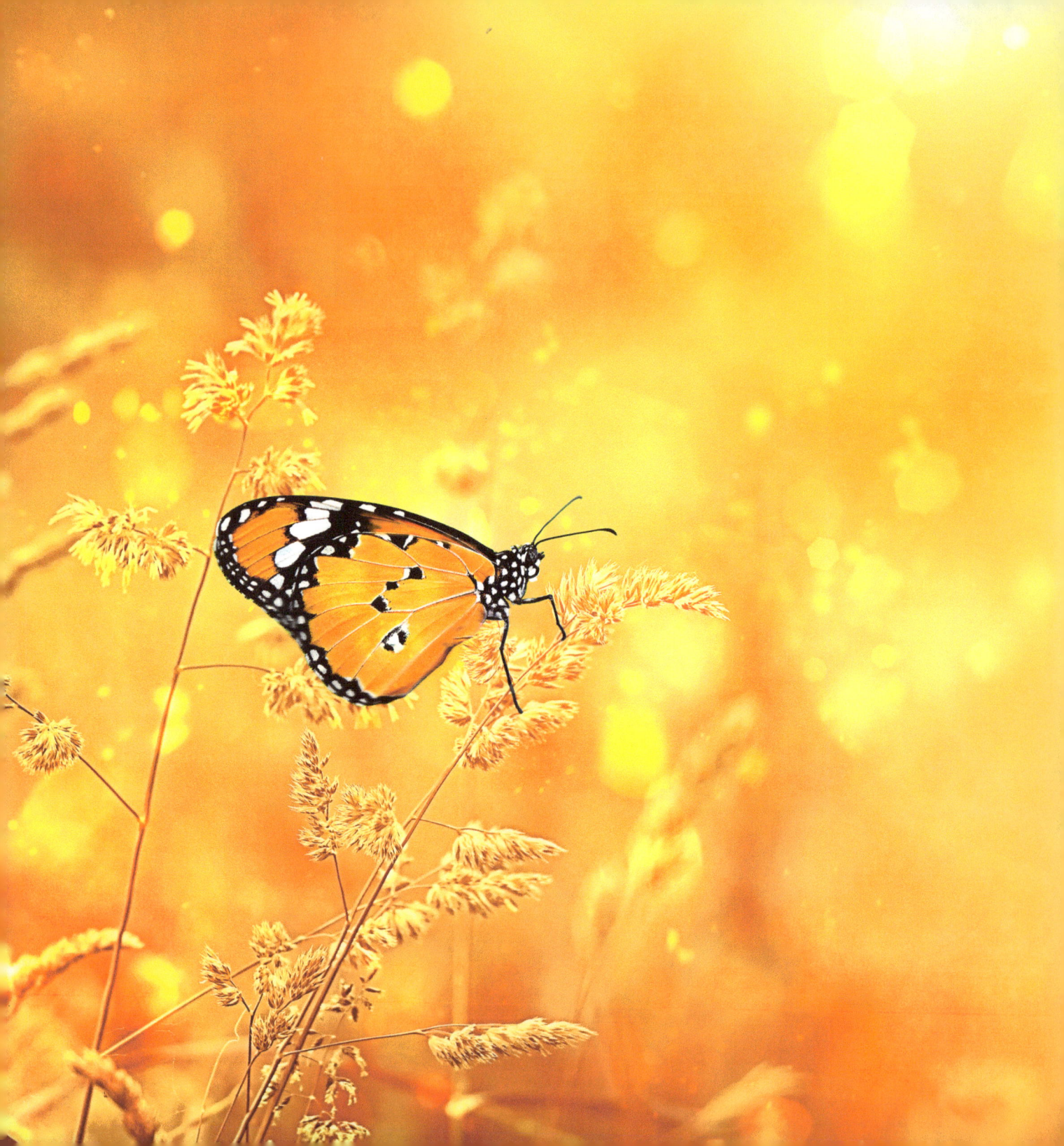

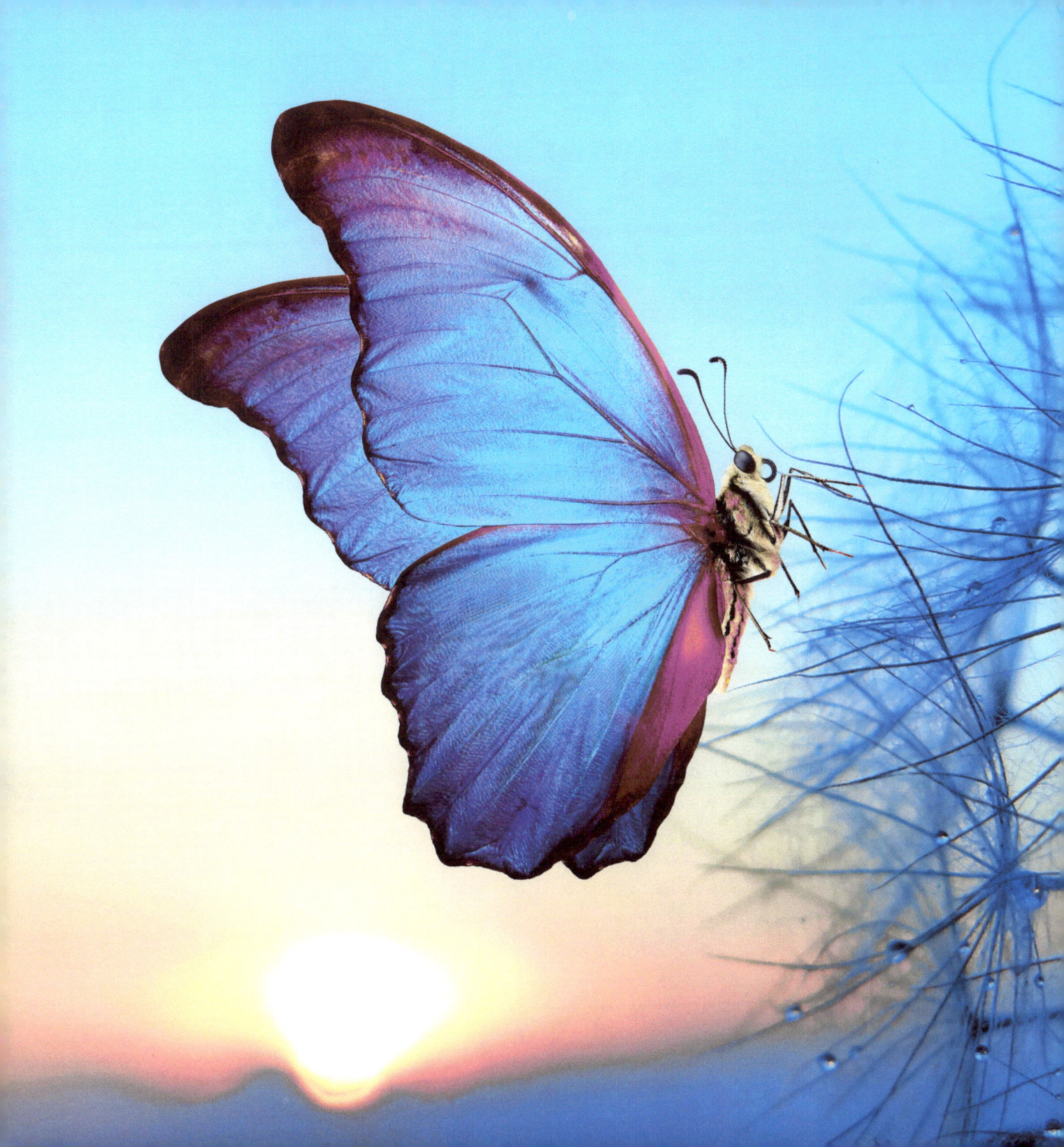

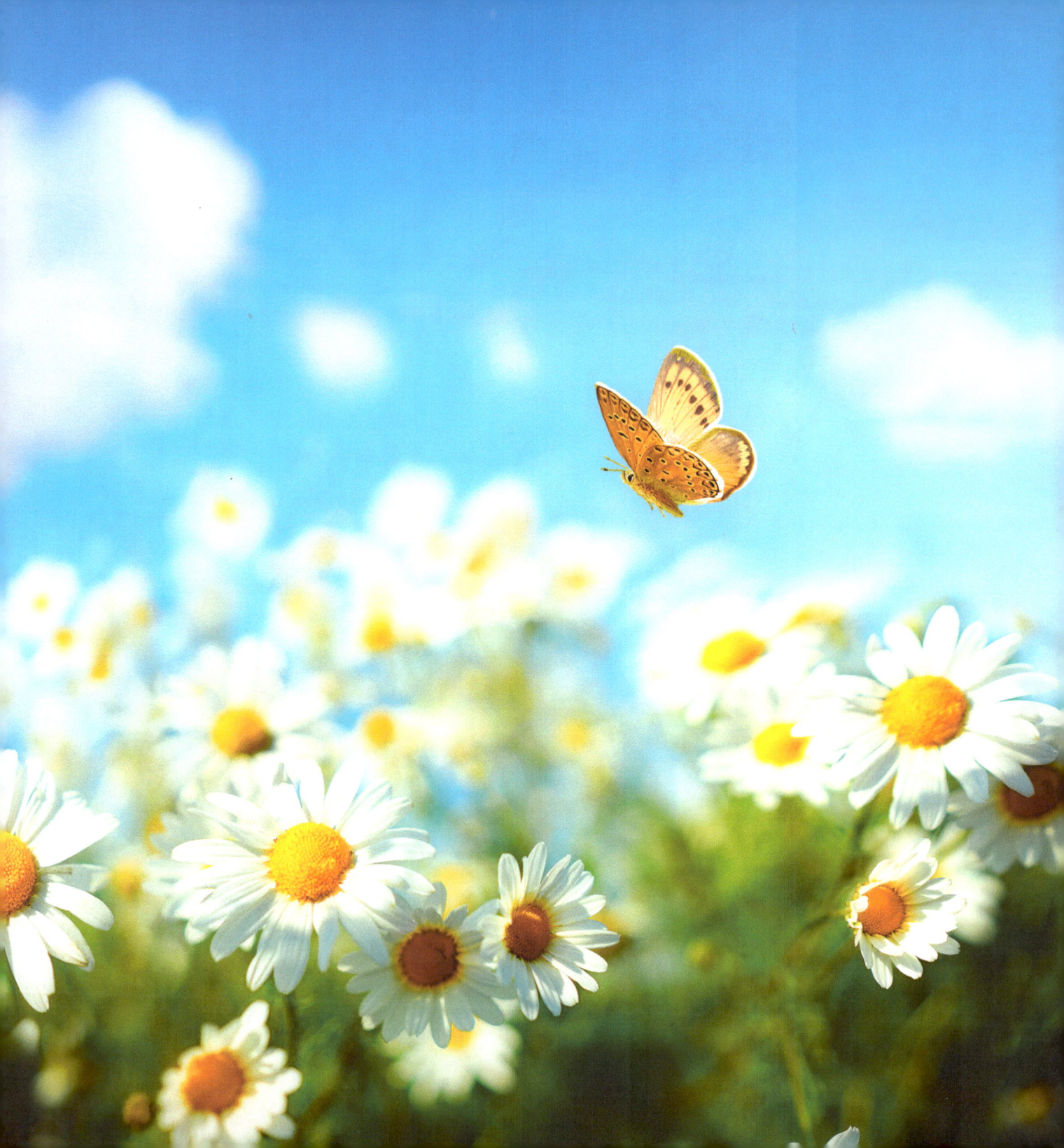

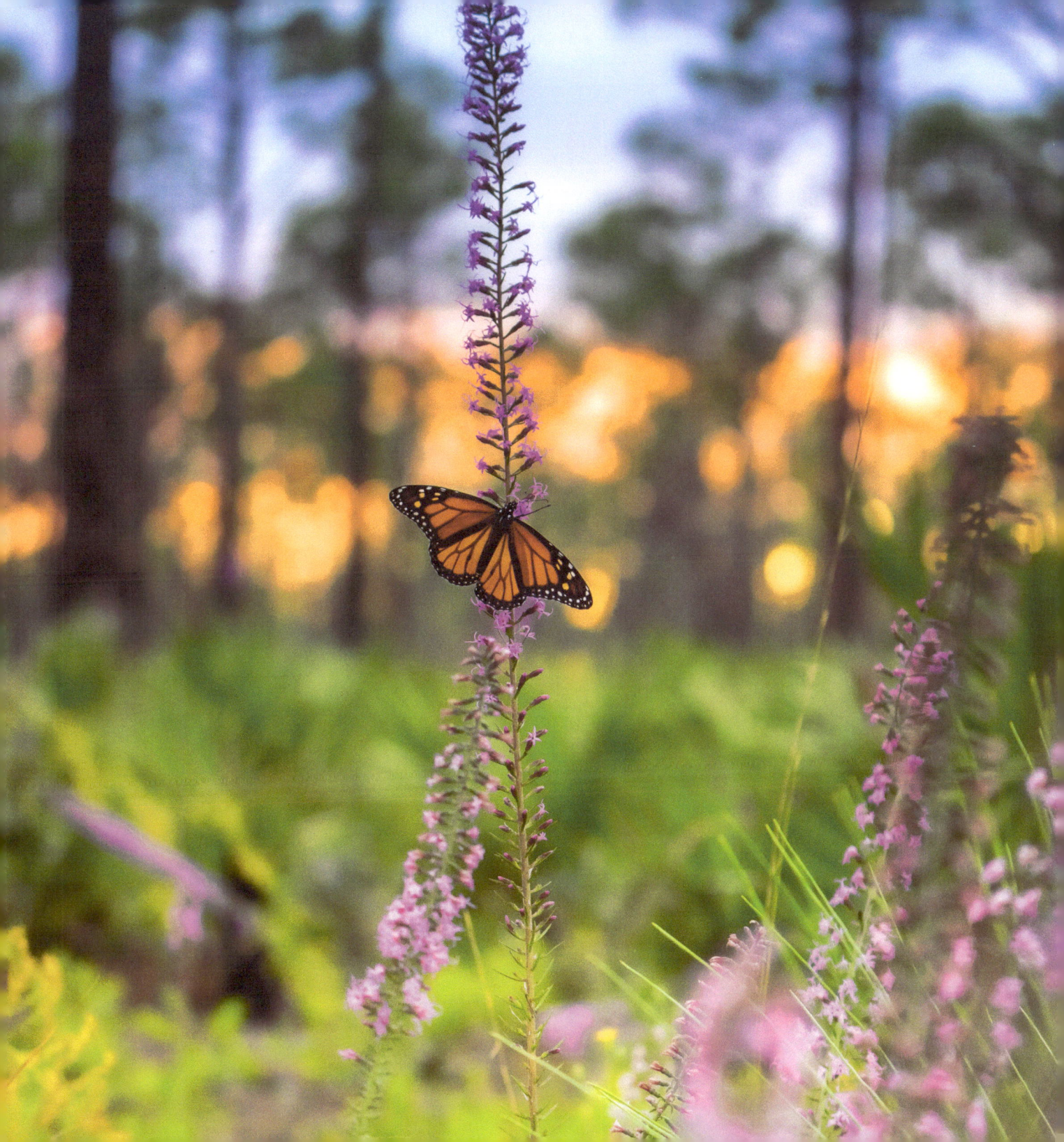

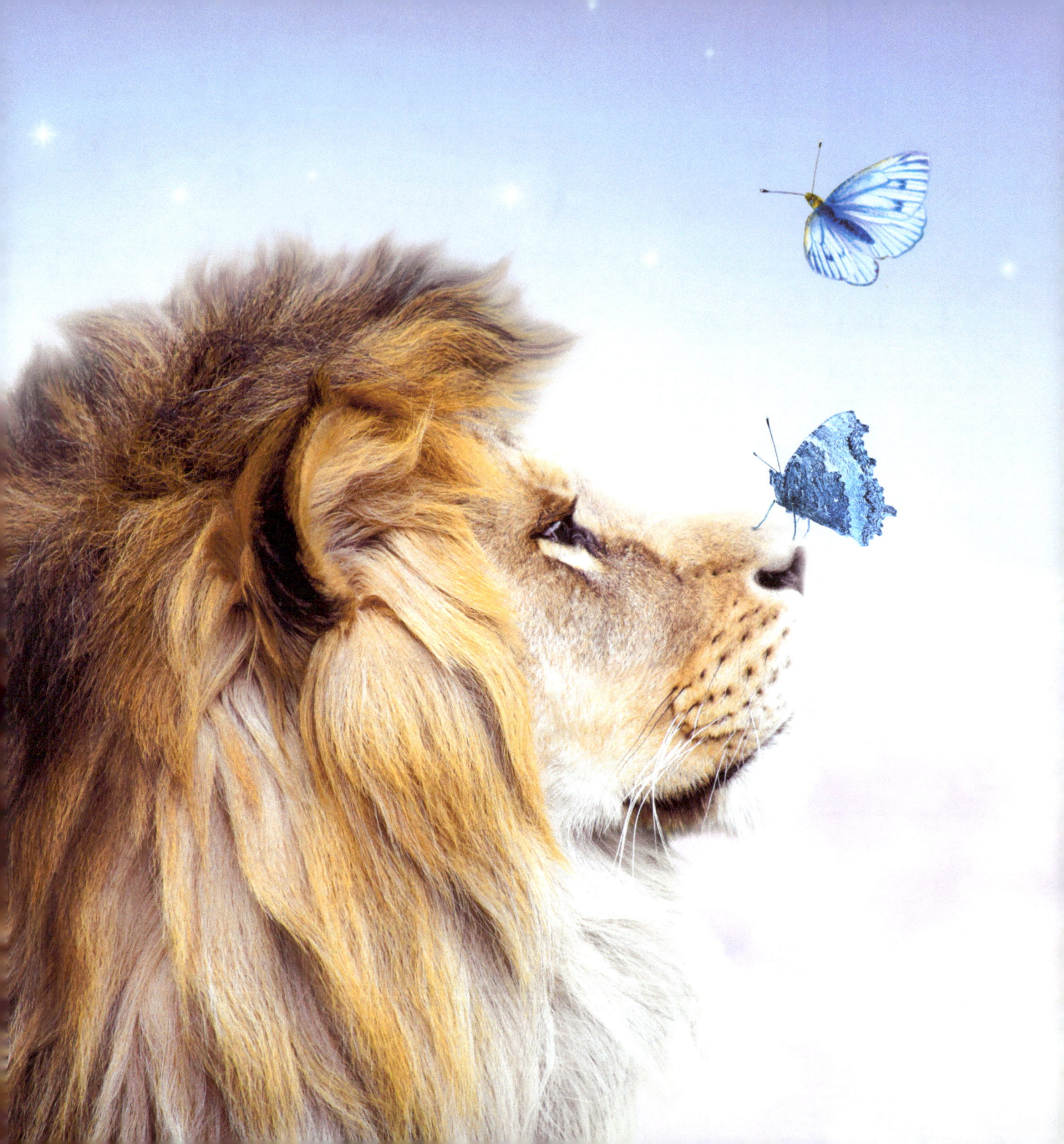

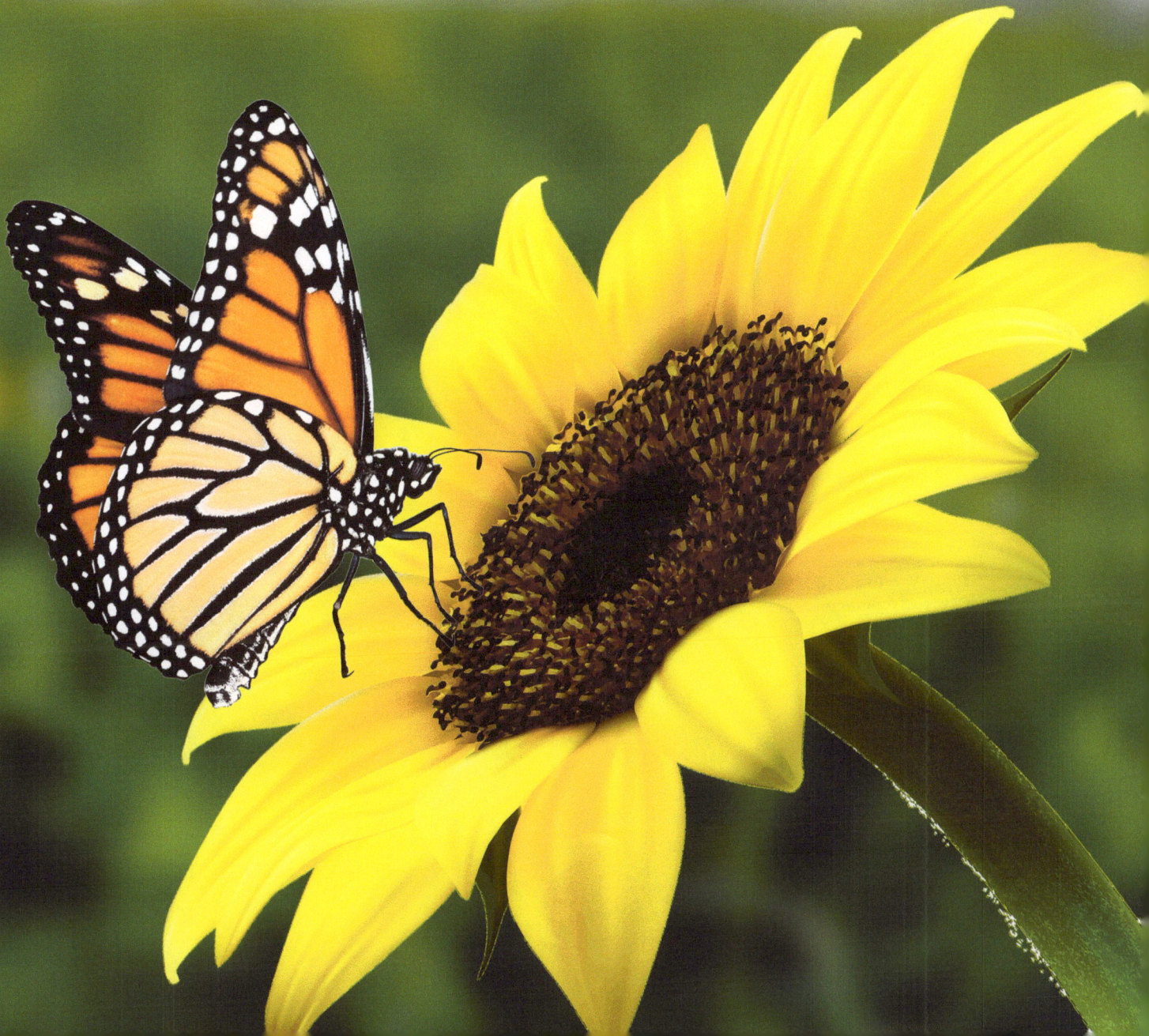

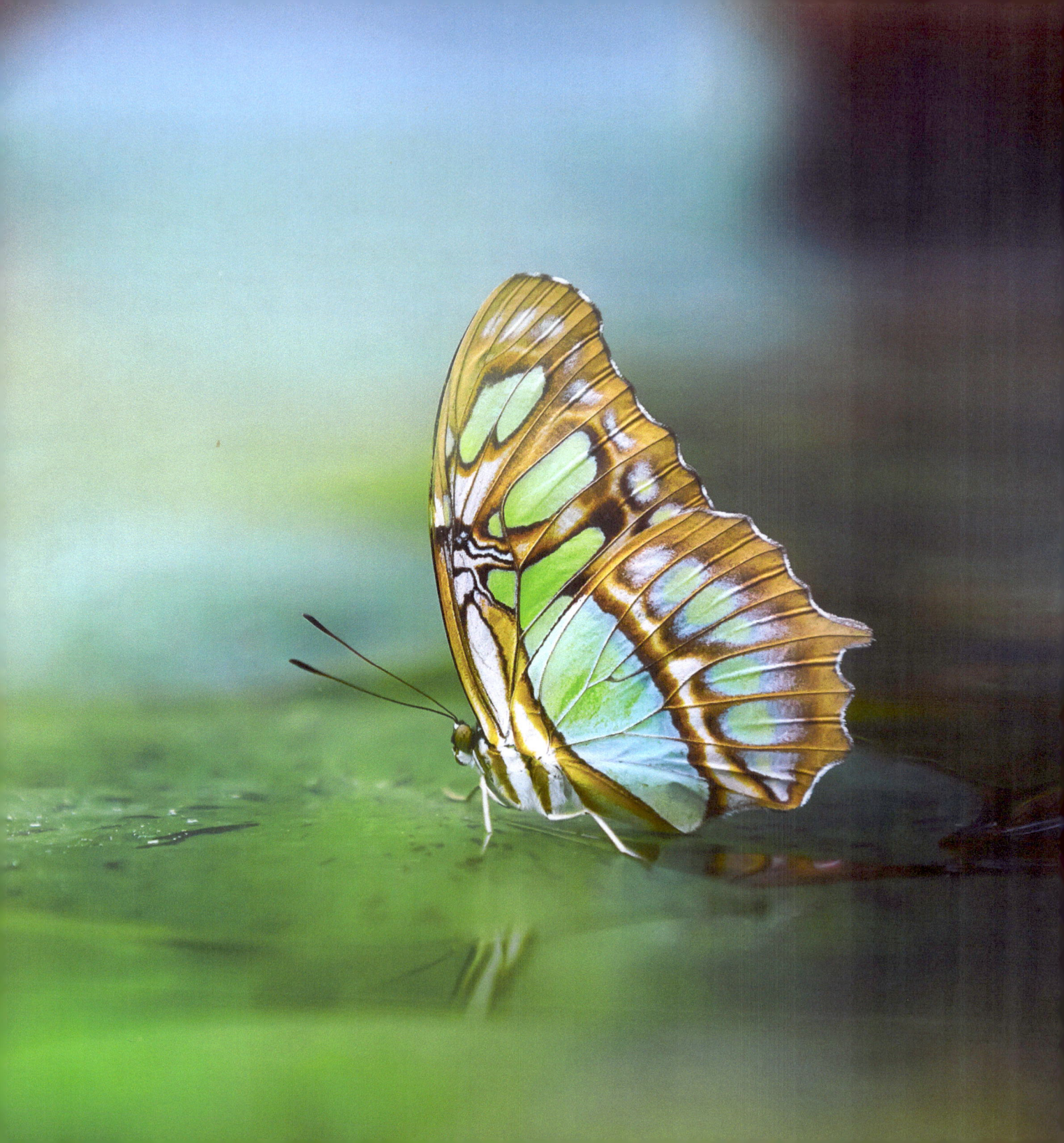

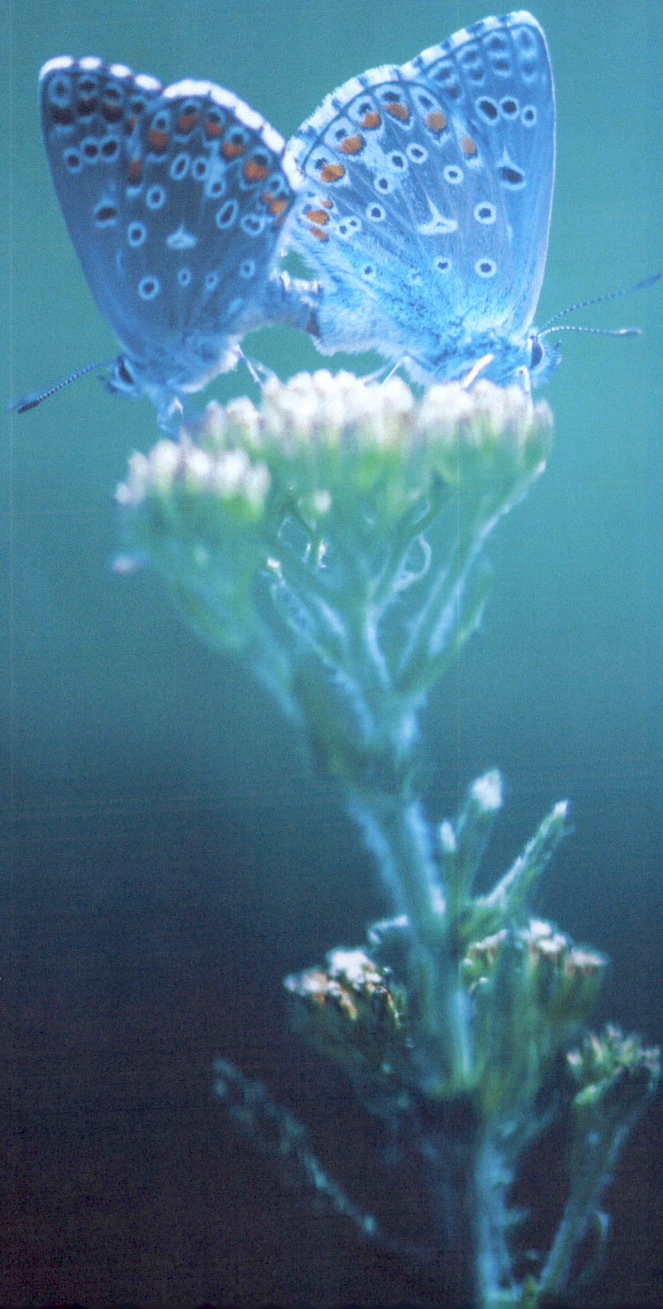

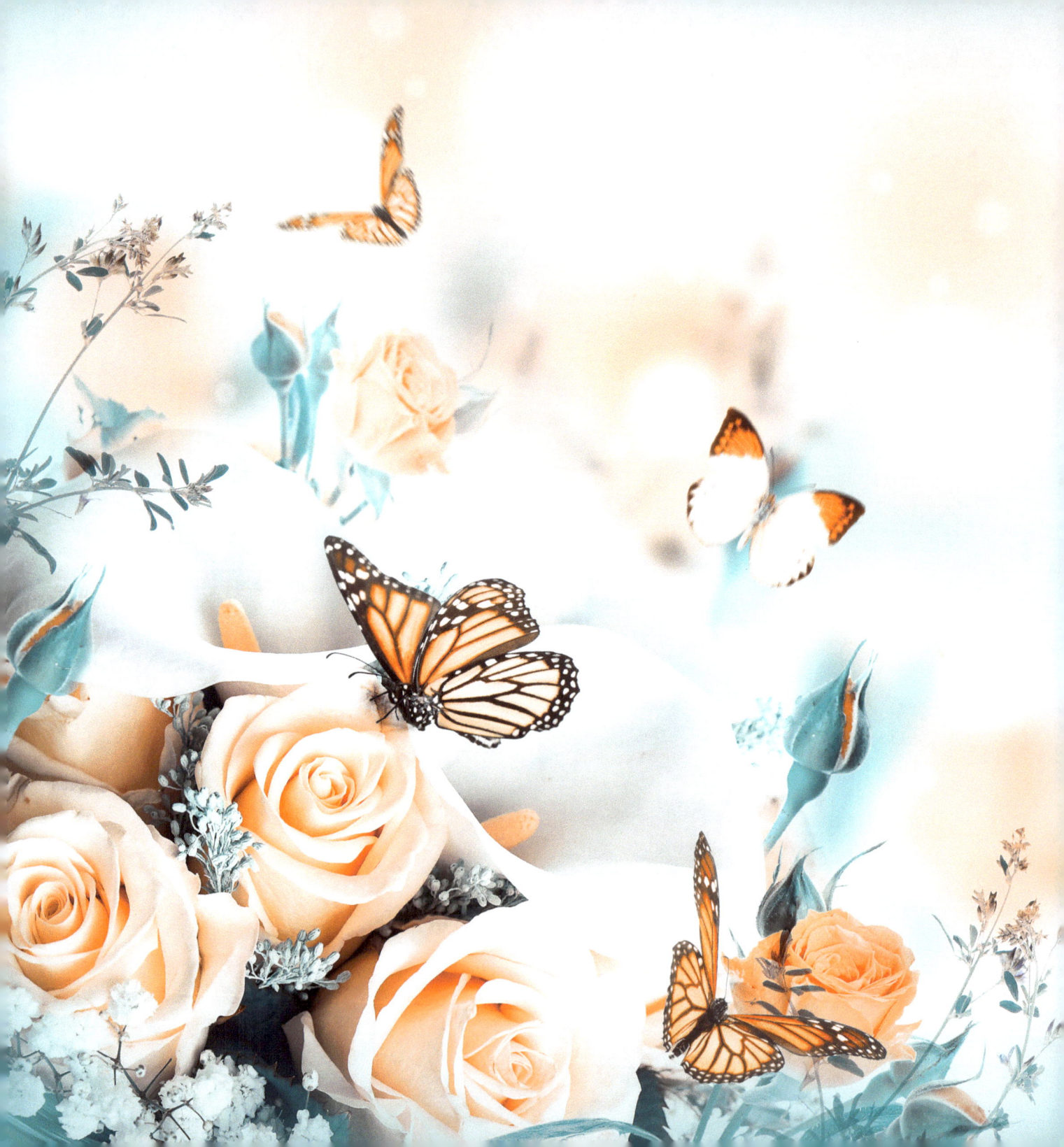

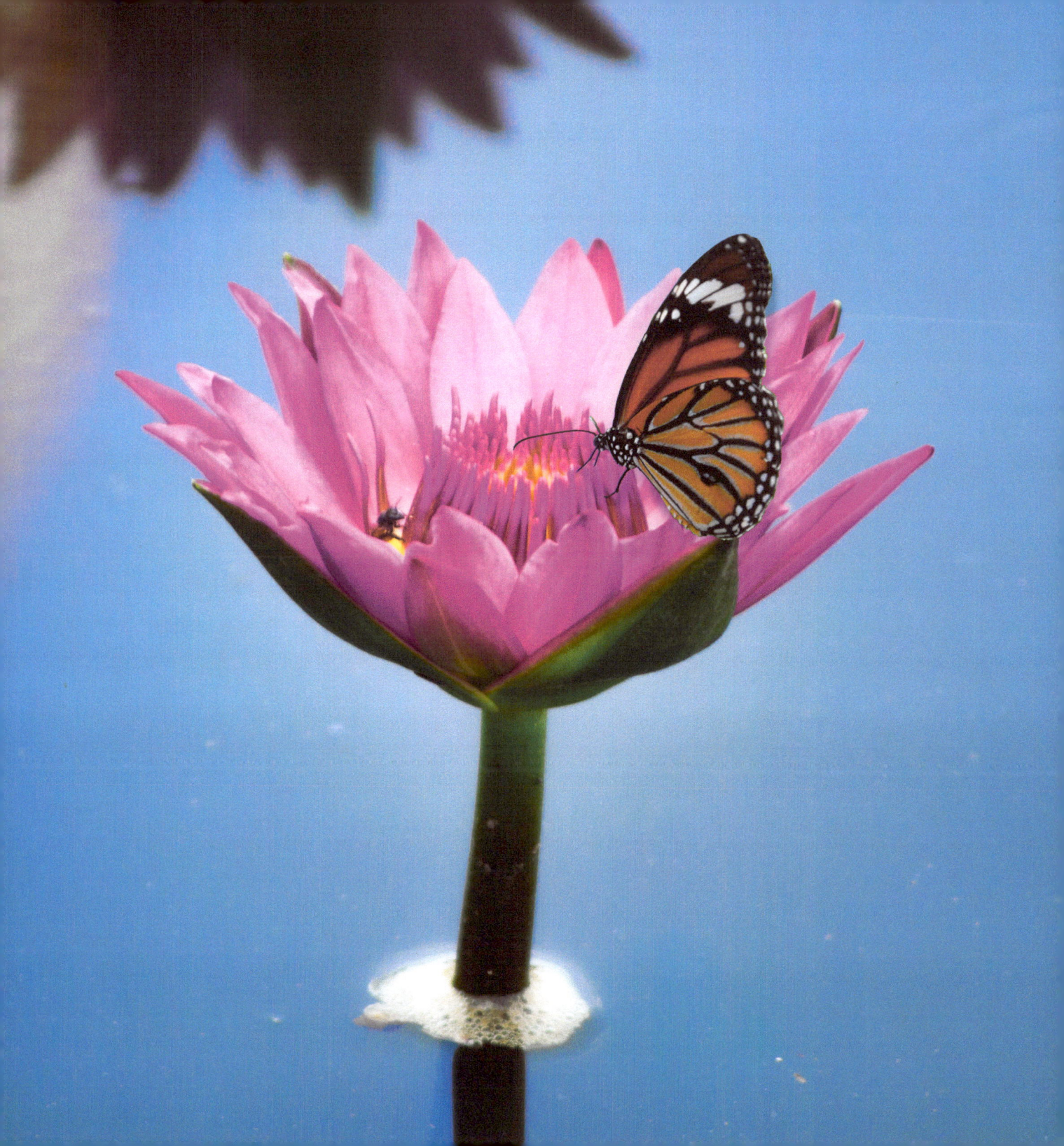

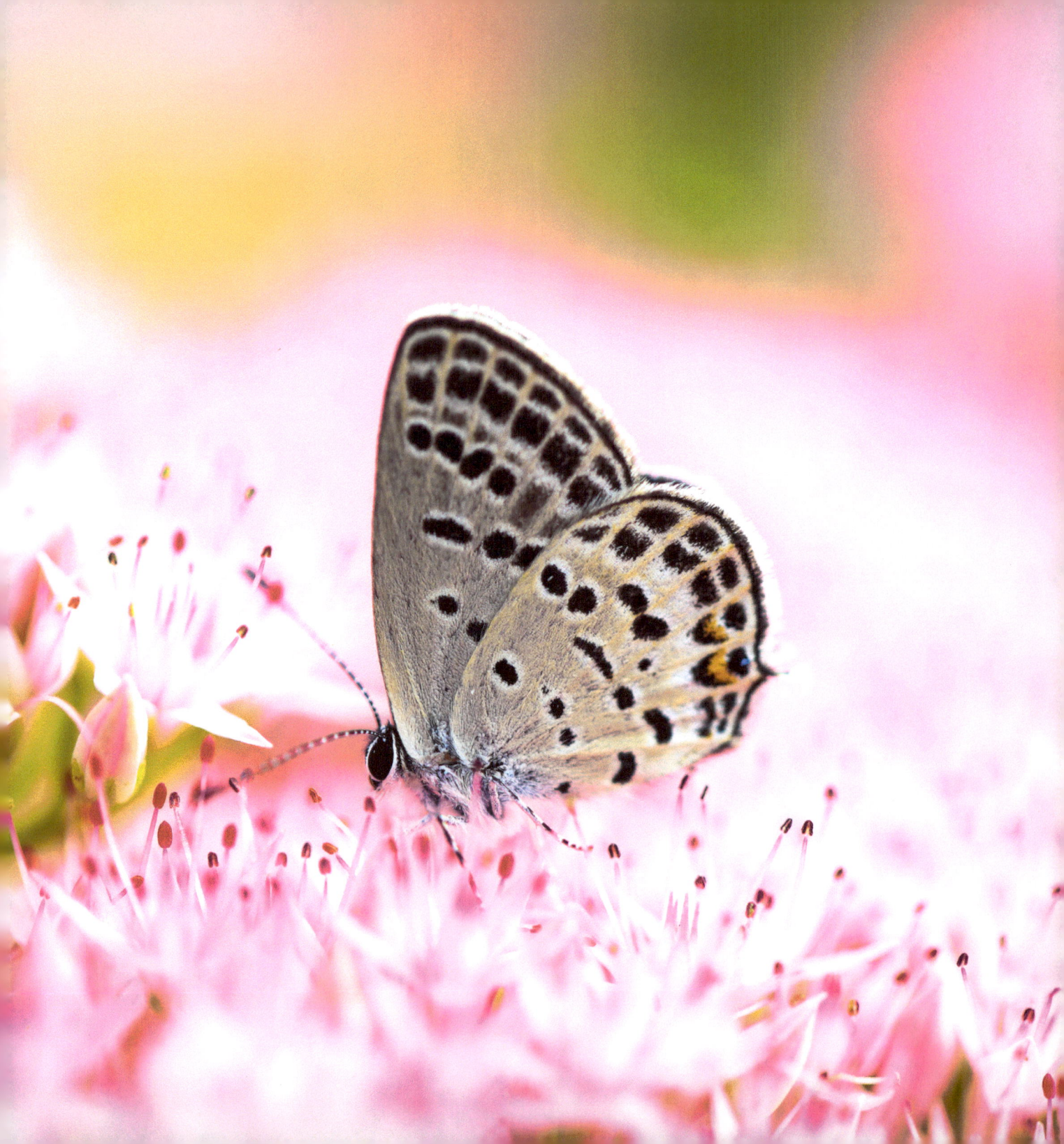

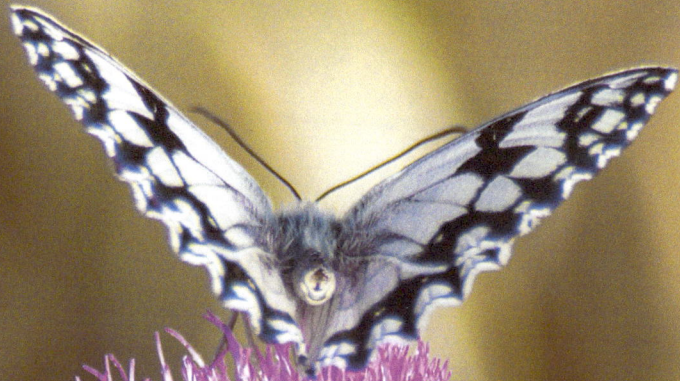

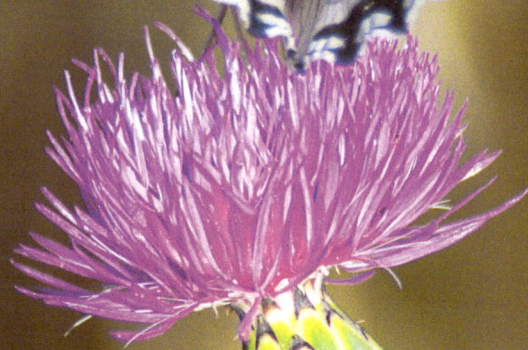

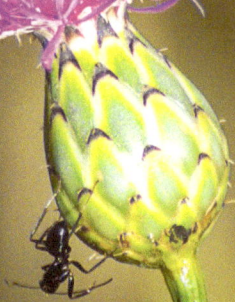

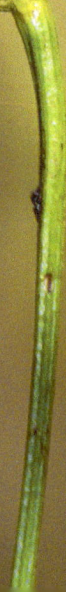

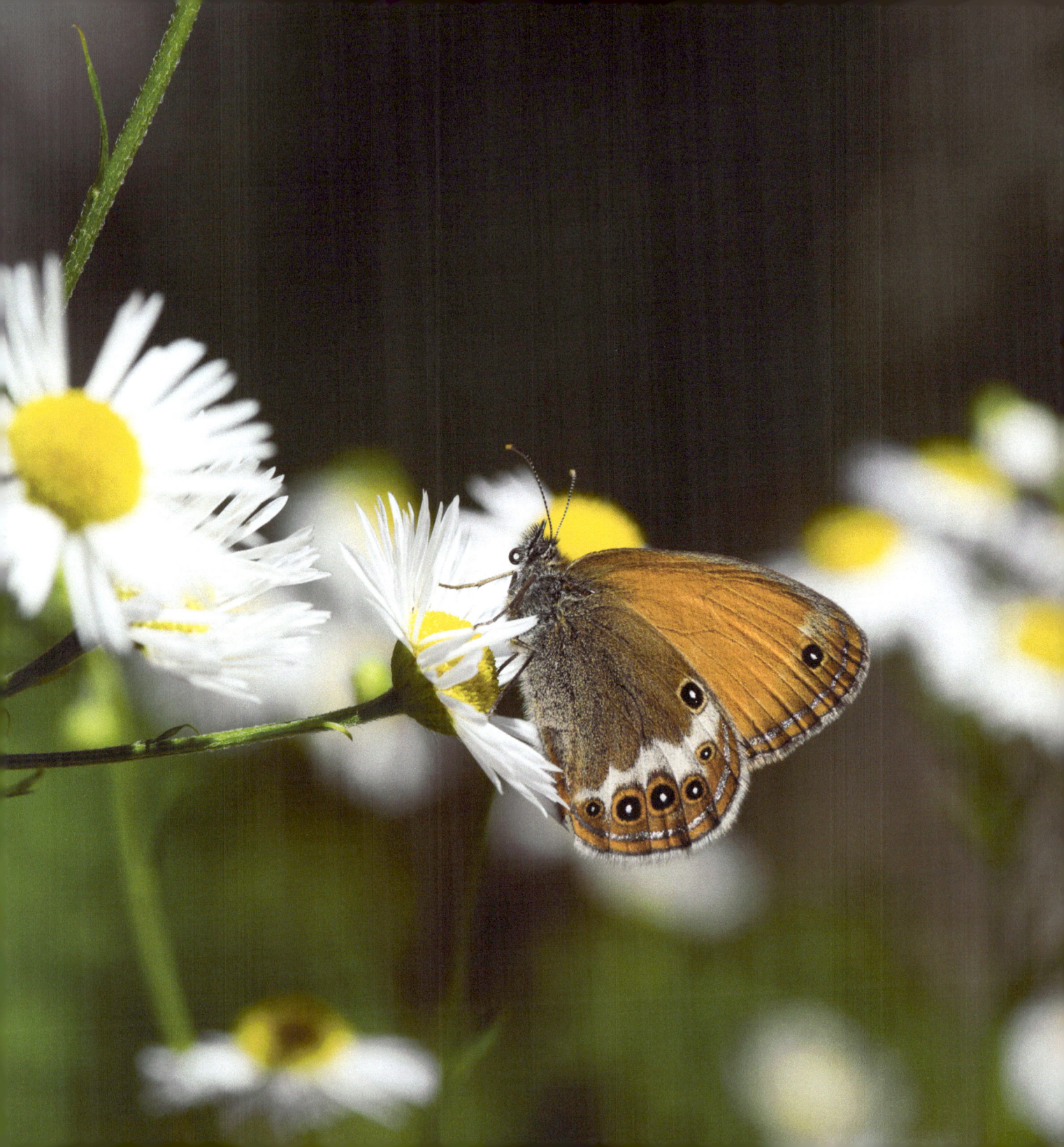

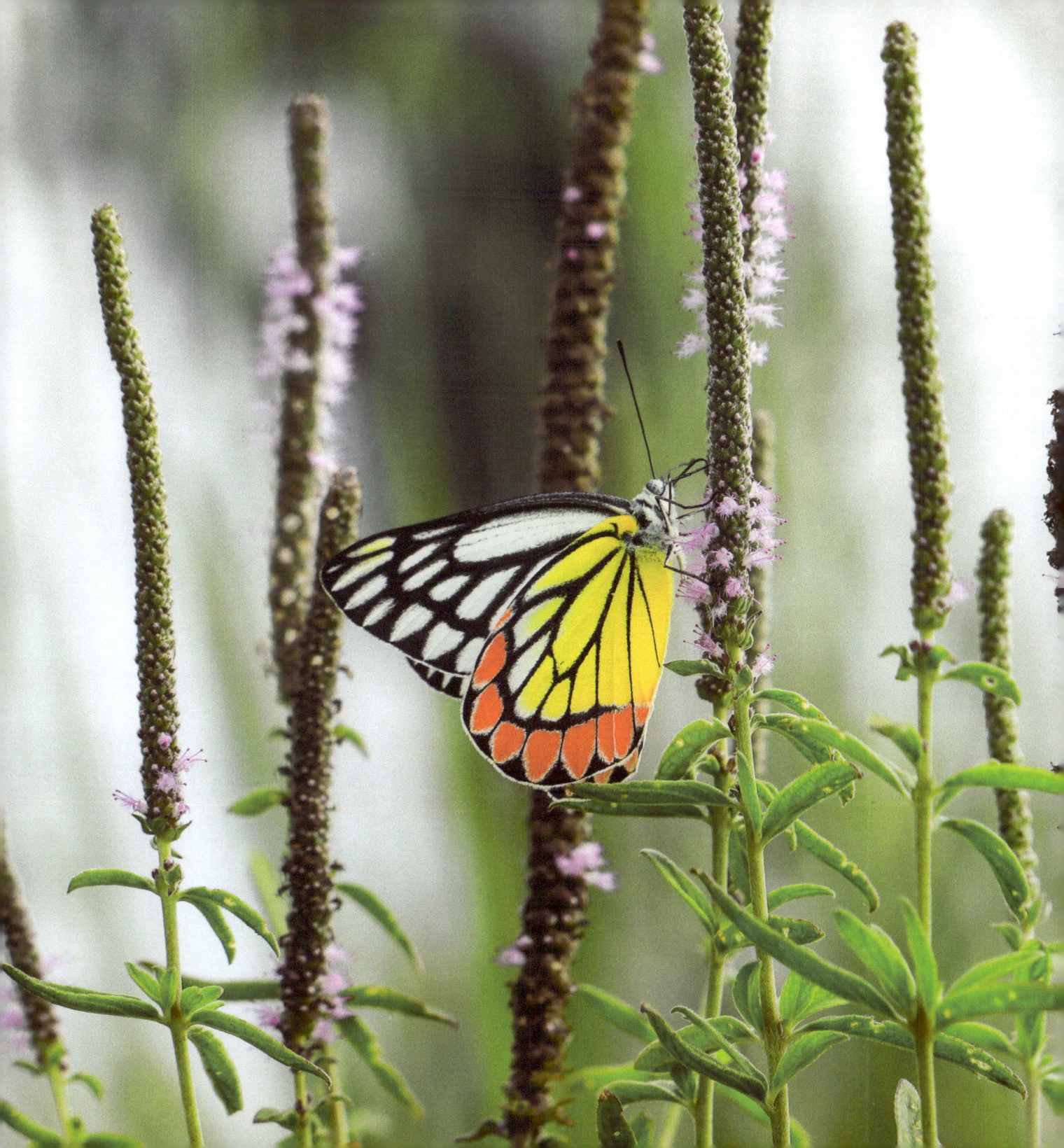

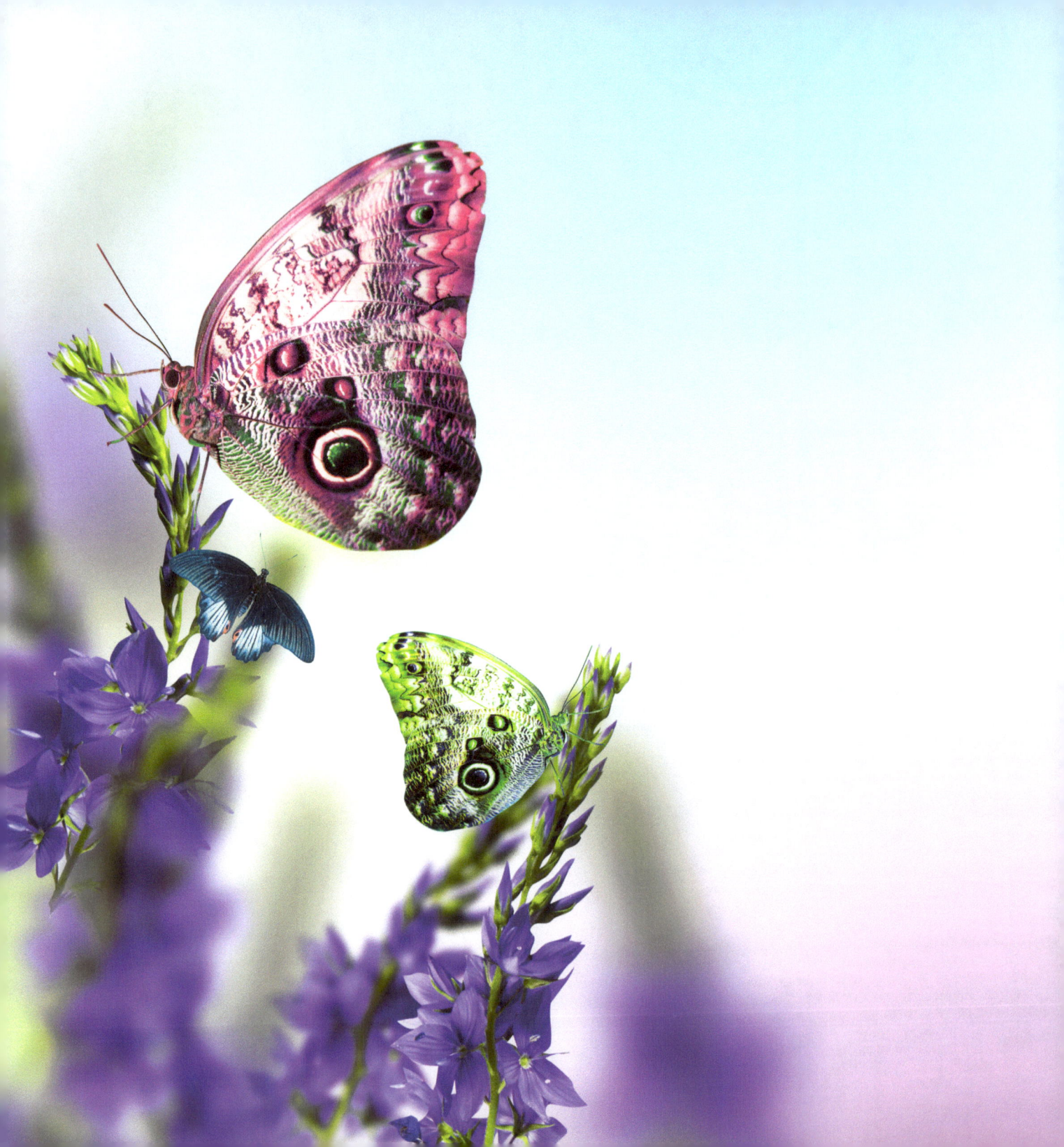

www.ingramcontent.com/pod-product-compliance
Lightning Source LLC
Chambersburg PA
CBHW061142030426
42335CB00002B/76